Timothy Richards Lewis /David Douglas Cunningham
The Fungus-Disease of India
A report of observations

SE**V**ERUS
Verlag

Lewis, Timothy Richards/Cunningham, David Douglas:
The Fungus-Disease of India. A report of observations.
Hamburg, SEVERUS Verlag 2011.
Nachdruck der Originalausgabe von 1875.

ISBN: 978-3-86347-128-6
Druck: SEVERUS Verlag, Hamburg 2011

Der SEVERUS Verlag ist ein Imprint der Diplomica Verlag GmbH.

Bibliografische Information der Deutschen Nationalbibliothek:
Die Deutsche Nationalbibliothek verzeichnet diese Publikation in der
Deutschen Nationalbibliografie; detaillierte bibliografische Daten sind
im Internet über http://dnb.d-nb.de abrufbar.

CONTENTS.

CHAPTER I.

THE NATURAL HISTORY OF PARASITIC FUNGI GENERALLY.

CHAPTER II.

THE EVIDENCE RECORDED IN FAVOUR OF THE FUNGAL ORIGIN OF THE MADURA FOOT-AND-HAND-DISEASE.

CHAPTER III.

A DESCRIPTION OF SPECIMENS ILLUSTRATIVE OF THE PALE VARIETY OF THE FUNGUS-DISEASE OF INDIA.

CHAPTER IV.

PHYSICAL CHARACTERS AND RELATIONS TO SURROUNDING
TISSUES OF THE MORBID PRODUCTS OF THE PALE VARIETY
OF THE DISEASE.

CHAPTER V.

PHYSICAL CHARACTERS AND INTIMATE NATURE OF THE RED
PARTICLES OCCASIONALLY ASSOCIATED WITH THE PALE
VARIETY OF THE FUNGUS-DISEASE OF INDIA.

CHAPTER VI.

A DESCRIPTION OF SPECIMENS ILLUSTRATIVE OF THE DARK
VARIETY OF THE FUNGUS-DISEASE OF INDIA.

CHAPTER VII.

PHYSICAL CHARACTERS AND RELATIONS TO SURROUNDING
TISSUES OF THE BLACK MATTER FREQUENTLY ASSOCIATED
WITH THE FUNGUS-DISEASE OF INDIA.

CHAPTER VIII.

CULTIVATIONS OF THE VARIOUS MORBID PRODUCTS OF THE
DISEASE.

CHAPTER IX.

LESSONS TO BE DERIVED FROM THESE CULTIVATION-EXPERI-
MENTS.

CHAPTER X.

CONCLUSIONS.

ILLUSTRATIONS.

FUNGUS-DISEASE OF INDIA.

CHAPTER I.

THE NATURAL HISTORY OF PARASITIC FUNGI GENERALLY.

THE importance of undertaking a series of systematic observations with a view to elucidate the nature of the connection between certain disease-processes and growths

Reasons for undertaking the study of the relation of fungi to disease.

of a vegetable character has for a long time been impressed upon us, and we have for several years past kept records of investigations bearing more or less directly on this subject. Hitherto, however, our reports on fungi and allied organisms have referred to the question of the actual presence of any such vegetations, not palpably adventitious, in connection with certain special diseases, and particularly with cholera. Having failed to satisfy ourselves of the existence of sufficient evidence to support the doctrine that any such growths are necessarily associated with these particular classes of disease, we decided on ascertaining, if possible, whether in the diseased conditions in which characteristic fungoid growths are known to exist beyond dispute, the latter are to be regarded as the actual cause of the particular malady. In undertaking this work we were aware that it was taking a step backward—treading the ladder a step lower down than that on which we commenced our work. We saw no alternative, however, but to do this, as personal observation had taught us that certain fundamental data, which we had originally taken for granted as established, were not entitled to such unreserved reliance. Some of these observations we now propose to detail.

We are desirous that it should be understood that
Not our intention to discuss purely botanical questions. it is not our intention to discuss the purely botanical questions which, though so intimately associated with phyto-pathological studies, belong, nevertheless, more to the province of the professional botanist than to that of the pathologist: such questions, for example, as the relation existing between fungi and algæ. The true character of the vegetations which occupy debatable land between fungi and algæ—aquatic fungi, *Achlya, Saprolegnia,* and the like—is of itself a question sufficiently difficult to occupy the undivided attention of botanical experts for years to come, so that we do not consider it necessary to offer any excuse for leaving such questions to those in whose province they lie, and restricting ourselves to their pathological bearings. We are the more inclined to this course, as there are, unfortunately, only too many examples on record of the great hindrance to the advancement of our knowledge of the causation of diseases which has been occasioned by pathologists and botanists having trespassed on each other's domains. This is an evil which it shall be our endeavour to avoid.

It will be convenient for many reasons to restrict
The term 'fungus' adopted as being the most convenient in describing epi- and endo-phytic growths. ourselves to the employment of one term whilst describing the particular vegetations under discussion; and as it is only very rarely that what, in the present state of our knowledge, are regarded as 'algæ' manifest truly parasitic proclivities, we shall refer to them as 'fungi' simply.

The opinion that fungi are endowed with the power
The influence of 'vitality' in limiting the spread of fungi. of inducing disease is not an unnatural one, seeing that they are the most constant of all the attendants on disease and decay. Their germs are known to be universally distributed, and were it not for the peculiar conditions required for their development, their depredations would be past conception. Fortunately, nature has fixed a

very potent barrier between a sporule and the organised material upon which it may chance to settle, and which, were it not for this barrier, it would speedily appropriate to its own use. This barrier is healthy life. It has yet to be shown that the living matter of the tissues of any animal, so long as it retains its vitality undiminished, is liable to succumb to the attacks of a fungus. Should a spore be brought into contact with bioplasm whose vitality is impaired, however, the changes in the latter which such impairment implies may be of a kind to transform it into most suitable pabulum for the nourishment of the former. The impairment of vitality may be due either to disease, or be a normal process, the result of age : whether the change be normal or abnormal matters little to the fungus—it grows and multiplies wherever it finds material exactly suited to it.

It is the less vitalized portions of animals that are prone to epiphytic attacks—portions which have little or no power of repair. Hence the epidermic tissues, the wing covers and articular plates of flies and other insects, branchial plates of fishes, and the like, are the parts on which fungi are most commonly found. In such cases the vegetable organisms do not attack the living material, but what has ceased to undergo any active nutritive changes and is virtually dead, excreted material. With regard to those instances in which it is known that fungi are associated with the existence of disease during life, it is far from proven in any single case that the disease was not present prior to the fungus. For example, it is most strongly maintained by many observers that it is only the sickly silkworm that is ever attacked by fungi, and that inoculation can only be effected after the worm has sickened.

There is another barrier to the unlimited development of fungi, although of less import so far as the growth of the mere vegetative portion of the fungus is concerned, and that is the adaptability of the soil for its nourishment. Even with regard to animal parasites this feature is particularly evident, not only with respect to the entozoa,

The nutritive requirements of fungi.

but epizoa also are limited to certain animals and even to certain defined areas of the body. This law applies as strictly with regard to fungi as to the higher plants; one spore will sprout and rapidly cover a surface with mould where another will not manifest the slightest indication of growth.

Some leaves become the hosts of certain fungi only— their entire surface being equally liable to attack; whereas it is only on a very limited area of other leaves that other species will develope at all. In Calcutta, for instance, the leaves of *Hibiscus rosæ sinensis*, at particular times of the year, almost invariably present a fungus on their surface, the growth of which is strictly limited to the point on the under surface, where the petiole enters the lamina of the leaf, and which does not spread beyond this spot notwithstanding the production of an abundant development of mycelium and sporular elements. It is evident that at this spot a peculiar secretion is present which furnishes suitable pabulum for the nourishment of the particular fungus.

Probability of certain plants producing secretions specially adapted to the growth of certain fungi.

As already mentioned, even some animals, just as in the case of the leaf, while in perfect health, appear to furnish a secretion which throughout life, and without detriment to their health, supports the growth of some particular fungus at a particular spot; and it is not improbable that the morbid secretions resulting from disease in others furnish the special pabulum necessary for the development of the particular kinds of fungi constantly forming so prominent a feature in the appearance of such animals both before and after death.

Probability of certain diseases producing secretions specially adapted to the growth of fungi.

Of animal tissues none are more frequently affected by fungi during life than the bodies of insects of various kinds; but whether the tissues are ever attacked during perfect health is, as already mentioned, a question still warmly disputed. This point, although it may appear, at first

Flies and insects attacked by fungi.

sight, to be of very trifling moment, is nevertheless of the utmost importance in estimating the nature and the extent of the influence which fungi exert on the production and maintenance of disease. The fact that the entire bodies of flies, beetles, bees, and such like, when affected with fungi, are found, when examined after death, to have been permeated through and through by mycelial threads, would be most significant were it known beyond doubt that the tissues in question were not diseased before the advent of the fungus—that the fungus did not follow the disease as the roots of a plant creep towards a stream.

Should it, however, be demonstrated that in any disease the growth of a fungus in a living subject can be limited not only to certain tissues, but to certain completely isolated portions of such tissues, the question would be very much simplified : such evidence would point to the dependence of the fungoid growths on some peculiar condition in those localised spots. It would, further, be evident that, however extensive, in some cases, the modification in the aspect and effects of the disease by the development of a fungus might be, the interpretation to be put upon the *rôle* of the latter in the malady must be in accordance with the fact that its development depended upon some previous change in the normal tissues.

The inferences which would be natural were isolated growths of fungi in the tissues demonstrated.

What our own conclusions are with regard to this matter in connection with the disease in which we have specially studied it, will be gathered from the following account of a series of observations extending over a period of several years. We have endeavoured to curtail the narrative as much as appears to be consonant with the desire that readers may be able to infer the extent and to know exactly the character of these observations, and thus be able to judge whether or not we have worked at the subject in such a way as to entitle us to form an independent opinion.

CHAPTER II.

THE EVIDENCE RECORDED IN FAVOUR OF THE FUNGAL ORIGIN OF THE
MADURA-FOOT- AND HAND-DISEASE, OR FUNGUS-DISEASE OF INDIA.

THE disease which we have selected as being the most

*The bibliography of
the fungus disease of
India.*

suitable for the purpose we had in view—the ' Fungus-disease of India' —has been investigated with the greatest diligence and care by Dr. H. Vandyke Carter of Bombay, to whom the profession is indebted for by far the fullest information it possesses with regard to the affection, and who certainly was the first to describe accurately the minute characters of the black particles frequently found in connection with it. His published observations date as far back as March 1860, since which period several communications have appeared from his pen.* These he has summarised and supplemented in a very able monograph on the subject published during the past year.†

Dr. E. W. Eyre also has written a concise description of the disease, as witnessed by himself (*Indian Annals of Medical Science*, No. XII, pp. 513 and 813, 1860). He mentions that Garrison-Surgeon Godfrey of Madras was the first to call attention to the affection, under the designation of "Tubercular disease of the foot," and that he published an account of some cases observed by him since 1844, in the *Lancet*, 10th June 1846. The malady has, therefore, been known to the profession for more than thirty years.

No special interest was, however, taken in the matter until Dr. Vandyke Carter, as already mentioned, the

---

* *Transactions of the Medical and Physical Society of Bombay*, vol.   VI, 1860.
  Ditto   ditto   vol. VII, 1860.
  Ditto   ditto   vol. VIII, 1862.
 Transactions of the Pathological Society of London,   vol. XXIV, 1873.
† " Mycetoma," or the Fungus-disease of India—London: J. and A. Churchill, 1874.

Reverend M. J. Berkeley,[*] and Mr. H. J. Carter, F. R. s.,[†] published the result of their personal observations. The papers of these distinguished observers were followed by those of many others, so that the bibliography of the disease at present occupies no inconsiderable space in our medical literature. Those of our readers who may desire further details on this point will find a careful *resumé* of the greater part of what has been written concerning the disease in Dr. Carter's valuable monograph. It will be sufficient for our purpose merely to refer, generally, to what the three writers above mentioned have written, more especially to the writings of Dr. Vandyke Carter and Mr. Berkeley, with whom chiefly rest alike the credit and the responsibility which is attached to the observations and the deductions which have been promulgated with regard to the disease.

According to Dr. Carter, the affection manifests
Varieties of the disease distinguished by Dr. Carter. itself under two forms, each presenting a different stage of the same disease: (1), the *black* or *melanoid*, and (2), the *pale* or *ochroid*, varieties. There is, further, a phase of the disease characterised by the presence in the tissues of pink granules, so that, practically, the malady has been described as presenting three varieties. Although the phase of the disease last mentioned is of rare occurrence, it is, nevertheless, of great significance in connection with the theory of the origin of the disease now commonly accepted—a view typified in the name "Mycetoma" given to it by Dr. Carter and adopted by the London Royal College of Physicians in its 'Nomenclature of Diseases.'

As far as external appearances go, the two leading forms have much in common. There
The Dark and the Pale varieties compared—External appearances. is considerable distortion of the foot or hand affected, an increase of size,

---

* Intellectual Observer, No. X, November 1862.
  Journal of Linnean Society, vol. VIII, p. 135, 1865.
† Annals and Mag. Nat. Hist., vol. IX, 1862.
  Journal of the Linnæan Society, vol. VIII, 1865.

more or less marked, in all directions; there are numerous, somewhat mammillated, apertures, communicating with cavities of various sizes and channels of various lengths in the subjacent tissues. The materials which escape through these apertures differ in the two forms: in the dark variety the fluid which oozes from the foot frequently contains brownish-black granules, in appearance not unlike the rougher description of gunpowder; whereas in the pale variety little particles, bearing a considerable resemblance to fish-roe, are very commonly seen.

On section also the state of the hard and soft tissues presents much in common:—(*a*) numerous lined cavities generally communicating with each other by means of sinuous channels; (*b*) softening and excavations, more especially of the tarsal and carpal bones, but frequently also involving the long bones; and (*c*) the packing of these cavities with a hard, dark substance in the black variety, and with a more or less soft, yellowish, fatty or gelatinous substance mixed with globular roe-like particles in the other.

Appearances presented by the two varieties on section.

It is with reference to the nature of these two substances, so different in appearance to the naked eye, that Dr. Vandyke Carter's observations and deductions are of such importance; not only of importance in relation to the particular malady in which these peculiar substances are found, but to that class of diseases—a class at present very large and still on the increase—whose *existence* and *extension* is attributed solely to the pernicious influence of vegetable parasites.

Intimate nature of the abnormal products.

Briefly stated, Dr. Carter describes the dark material in the first variety of the affection as consisting almost entirely of a fungus in its sclerotial form, *i. e.,* one of the 'resting' states common to fungi and somewhat analogous to the 'resting' states of perennial plants—examples of which are furnished by bulbs and tubers of various kinds. The substance found filling the cavities in the pale variety is considered to be indicative of an advanced stage of the disease due to "a change—seemingly a degeneration—" of the darkened masses.

The fact that a pink mould has been developed in connection with specimens of both varieties has served as a link between the dark and the pale material; and this link has, so to speak, been completed by the circumstance that Dr. Carter has observed a case of the disease—practically forming, as before mentioned, a third variety, in which a pink coloration of the tissues, associated with innumerable pink particles—'fungus-bodies,' were its characteristic features. Here, therefore, we seem to have the key to the arch which sustains the hypothesis that the Madura-foot and hand-disease is originated and propagated by means of a peculiar fungus.

The Pink variety of the disease.

It is consequently of importance that all who desire to form a correct estimate of the value of so important and popular a doctrine—of importance were it only because of its popularity—and absolutely incumbent on such as by their writings promulgate views based, as far as the human subject is concerned, almost entirely on this peculiar malady, to examine this particular point closely. To the best of our knowledge, the following particulars comprise all that have been published with regard to the pink mould and the pink particles. With regard to these two sets of observations, it may be noted that, in the first instance, attention was arrested by the occurrence of pink particles comparable to "red-pepper grains" in the diseased tissue, accompanied by some pink staining.

The various observations recorded regarding the pink mould—'Chionyphe Carteri.'

Some time subsequently it was observed that a pink or crimson coloured mould had developed on separate specimens of the ochroid variety on two different occasions, and on particles of it placed in boiled rice-paste :—(1) on the exposed portion of a foot which had been macerating in water for eighteen months—the growth extending

The pink mould developed in connection with the Pale variety.

"even to the sides of the bottle;" (2) on a preparation which "had been put into a bottle with some fresh spirit" for preservation about two months previously: the part of the specimen which was above the surface of the fluid, owing to the evaporation of the spirit, acquired "a red tinge and soon after there appeared a thick layer of crimson mould;" and (3) in connection with some soft particles from a foot which had been placed in some boiled rice-paste a day after amputation: ten days afterwards buff and green moulds were observed, and a few days later a red tint was distinguishable, and stained filaments were traced to the particles.

A similar mould was obtained on four occasions in connection with fragments of black particles obtained from specimens of the dark or melanoid variety:—

The pink mould developed in connection with the Black variety.

(1). Some of these particles from a newly amputated foot were mixed with a little *cotton soil* ‘moistened with animal juices’ and kept for two years and nine months unopened. It was then observed that a thin reddish film had appeared on the still moist surface like that noticed on the salt pans in the marshes near Bombay.

(2). During the same period similar fresh particles, obtained from the same source as in the foregoing experiment, were placed on rice-paste and set aside in a corked bottle. This preparation also remained unchanged for nearly three years, ‘when, on opening the bottle and removing its contents into an open glass-cell, a *red mould* speedily made its appearance and spread luxuriantly: it had not, however, a clear connection with the fungus particles, but seemed to spring up independently of them upon the rice wherever this was exposed to the air.’

(3). Black particles were taken directly from another foot and placed in some moist ground rice. About six months afterwards a reddish tinge, passing on to crimson, was observed on the rice starch. ‘ *The black particles have remained unchanged* to all appearance, and the red stains do not surround them, but may spring up unconnectedly.’ (The italics are ours.)

(4). A set of three experiments was undertaken:—
(a) black particles and rice-paste, (b) rice-paste only, and
(c) black particles which had been kept dry in a box
for two or three years (mixed with rice-paste ?).

When examined within a month, the first was unchanged; the second, i. e., the rice-paste alone, presented
a suspicious reddish tinge in one part; and the third
was covered with a pink growth which grew 'equally
and spread everywhere, but its commencement had no
more apparent connection with the unaltered black
masses than in the other cases.'

A fifth series was undertaken, but as the specimens
were lost, details have not been given.

With regard to these observations, Dr. Carter writes
that at first he did not appreciate the significance of
this pink tinted growth until he had learnt Mr. Berkeley's
opinion that the peculiar mould was 'the perfect condition of the species.'

Mr. H. J. Carter made somewhat similar observations, and both observers communicated their results to
the Revd. Mr. Berkeley, who, as being the most experienced and distinguished mycologist in England, was
of all persons the most likely to be able to throw light
on the nature of the growth.

Mr. Berkeley also undertook some cultivation-experiments with material obtained from
The Revd. Mr. Ber-
keley's observations
regarding the pink
mould.
Bombay—Dr. Vandyke Carter supplied some alcohol-preserved speci-
mens, and Mr. H. J. Carter some fragments of the
material preserved in dried rice-paste. No peculiar
growth was developed in connection with the former,
but a pink mould appeared on some rice-paste to which
some of the dried fragments had been added. Although
the growth of this mould did not proceed sufficiently
far to bring all its fruit to perfection, still, taking into
consideration the experience gained by the observers in
Bombay as well as his own, Mr. Berkeley felt himself
justified in pronouncing the mould to be new to science.
Though having many points in common with *Mucor*, it,
nevertheless, did not accurately coincide with all the

characters of that genus, but approached more nearly to the genus *Chionyphe*—every hitherto known species of which had only been observed to grow on melting snow. This pink mould was consequently added to the list of species of this genus and named *Chionyphe Carteri*.

As already intimated, it is not our intention to discuss the purely botanical phase—the phase which Mr. Berkeley naturally restricts himself to—but with regard to the assumed relation of this pink mould to the disease under consideration, the opportunity may be taken of pointing out here (1) that it was observed to grow without any appreciable connection with the black particles—the only substance associated with the malady in which the existence of fungoid elements has been definitely established; (2) that these particles themselves were, on every occasion, found to be wholly unchanged; and (3) that the pink mould grew as luxuriantly in connection with preparations which had been preserved in spirit as in connection with specimens of the morbid tissues which had not been subject to the influence of any preservative fluid.

CHAPTER III.

A DESCRIPTION OF SPECIMENS ILLUSTRATIVE OF THE PALE VARIETY
OF THE FUNGUS-DISEASE OF INDIA.

THE materials forming the subject of examination
were derived from entire preparations of both upper
and lower extremities affected by the disease, and
from numerous smaller specimens of the morbid tissues
from other cases. Considering the rarity with which
the disease attacks the upper extremity, we were for-
tunate in obtaining two excellent specimens in which
it was so localised. Taken together, the specimens
presented a series of typical examples of various
degrees of both the so-called pale and dark varieties
Materials examined.   of the disease, while one of them
afforded an abundant supply of the
peculiar red particles which are only very rarely found
in association with it—in fact, there appears to be only
one well authenticated case hitherto recorded—so that
we believe that we have had what may be regarded as
very fair opportunities for the study of the morbid appearances present, and of the lesions and pathological
changes affecting the tissues.

It is a matter of regret to us that we have had no
opportunity of studying the disease during life owing
to its extreme rarity in Calcutta—apparently it is not
endemic in this part of India, and consequently only
presents itself in the form of isolated imported cases.
We hope, however, that we may yet be able to complete our observations in this respect at some future
period in one or other of the endemic areas of the disease, for we feel that the careful study of the specimens
which have been at our disposal have rendered us
much better prepared for the clinical study of the
disease and the investigation of the conditions under
which it is developed than we could otherwise have
been.

We owe the materials which we have examined to the kindness of Dr. Cornish, the Sanitary Commissioner for Madras; Dr. Gamack, Civil Surgeon of Madura; Dr. Mark Robinson, at present acting for Dr. Gamack; Dr. Kenneth McLeod; Dr. Downie, Ulwar; and to the Civil Surgeon of Cuddapah; all of whom have, from time to time, either themselves supplied us with valuable specimens, or have induced others to do so. We wish, also, specially to acknowledge the obligation which we are under to Dr. McConnell, the Professor of Pathology in the Calcutta Medical College. He has not only aided us by supplying us with numerous specimens of the disease, but has placed the valuable collections in the Pathological Museum under his care at our disposal for purposes of examination and comparison.

The amount and variety of the labor involved in working out the subject has been considerable. Not only has it been necessary carefully to study the condition of the tissues and the nature of the morbid materials present in the various forms under which the disease presents itself, but a close examination of other *Nature of the investigations.* morbid tissues and products in other diseases affecting similar anatomical regions has had to be undertaken, together with a study of the nature and properties of various natural and artificial oleaginous compounds and concretions; and numerous and varied attempts at cultivation of the morbid materials, with study of the resultant organisms and of the effects of re-agents on them and other vegetable growths.

We take up the consideration of the Pale or Ochroid variety of the disease first as, in many ways, less obscure and complicated in character than that in which the black coloring of the morbid material forms such a *Reasons for beginning the report with a description of observations on the Pale variety of the disease.* striking and characteristic feature. It will, perhaps, be best in the first place to give a brief description of the appearances presented by some of the specimens which we have examined, and subsequently to consider the common features occurring in them all and, apparently, essentially connected with the disease. We shall then be in a position to state our views in regard to the pathology of the affection, together with the grounds on which these are based.

SPECIMEN I.—This consisted of a foot and ankle. The foot was much thickened, especially towards the ankle, and was straightened on the latter so as to point in a manner resembling that in cases of *Talipes equinus*. The toes presented much less distortion and tendency to be turned upwards on the foot than is, in our experience, usually the case in specimens of the disease. The general appearance of the specimen is shown in the accompanying woodcut (Fig. 1).

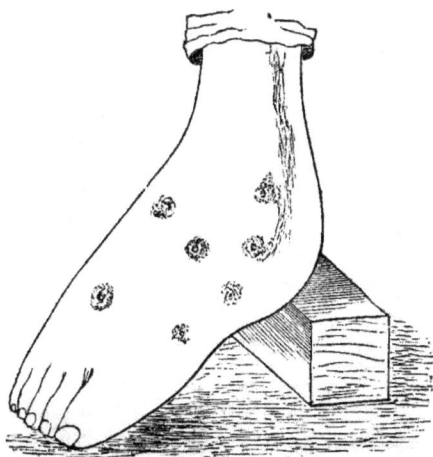

Fig. 1.—Outline sketch of a specimen of the Pale Variety of the Fungus-Disease of India.

Numerous openings surrounded by raised margins, or opening on the summits of elevated tuberculations, were present on both upper and under surfaces of the foot. They communicated with channels lined with smooth membranous tissue and leading into the substance of

the foot. On making a section, the knife passed readily
through the tarsal and metatarsal
bones and through the lower ex-
tremity of the tibia. All these bones were extremely
soft and opened-out in texture. The degree of softening
varied in different places ; in many it had proceeded so
far as to render the bones quite spongy and so friable as
to be easily broken up under the finger-nail even on
the surface, and in some places the softening had proceeded to such an extent as to replace the bone-texture
entirely by a soft greasy pulp. In those cases in which
the softening was only partial, the outline of the bones
could yet be traced, but in other places the latter were
quite indistinguishable from the surrounding degenerated tissues. One or two examples of cavities in the
substance of the bones were also present,—smooth, and
lined by a distinct membrane. Close to several of the
articulations there was some slight roughness of the surfaces of the bones. The muscular and tendinous
structures of the foot were well preserved and apparently
unaffected by the disease; but there was a general
thickening of the areas normally occupied by fat and
connective tissue, and all the structures were much
obscured by the extreme abundance of fatty matter present. There were numerous cavities in the substance
of the foot, lined by smooth membrane and containing oily and fatty material. Some of them were
quite isolated, but others communicated with one another, and with the exterior, by means of the channels
previously alluded to. One cavity of large size was
situated immediately above the metatarsal bones; it was
lined by a gelatinous pulp of orange yellow colour and
contained a large quantity of oily matter.

The extremely oily condition of all the tissues was
most remarkable, the bones were re-
duced to mere masses of soft fat pene-
trated and supported by remains of the osseous tissue;
and it was impossible to touch the preparation without
smearing the fingers, knives, and other instruments with
a thick coating of greasy oil, while the spirit in which it

Description of Speci-
men I—Greasy aspect
of the preparation.

Abundance of oily
matter in the tissues.

was preserved was covered with a thick layer of large yellow oil globules. The oily matter was throughout generally more or less fluid, but in some places both in the bones and soft tissues there was an abundance of distinct small glistening particles of a white colour and composed of dense radiating masses of acicular fat crystals. Nowhere was there the slightest indication of the presence of any brown or black matter, or of any peculiar substance save the profusion of oily matter. The amount of thickening in the masses of connective tissue rendered it probable that a certain amount of elephantoid condition had coincided with the pathological changes proper to the disease under consideration, and the distortion of the foot was in this case to be ascribed in great part to this, although, no doubt, the action of the tendons and muscles on the softened fatty bones also contributed to cause the distortion.

Careful microscopical examinations were made of all Microscopic examination. the tissues and materials present, but in no case did they afford the faintest evidence of the presence of any fungal or fungoid bodies, or of anything save degenerations of the normal elements of the tissues.

SPECIMEN II.—This preparation, which has already been referred to by Dr. Fayrer in his "Clinical and Pathological Observations in India," consisted of a foot and ankle.

The foot was much distorted: there was great Description of Specimen II. thickening anteriorly, and the toes were elevated and curved upwards from their bases. Numerous crater-like openings on the surface communicated with channels, lined by smooth membrane and leading into the interior of the foot. It was carefully divided longitudinally, the knife passing readily through the bones of the tarsus. As may be observed in the accompanying figure of the specimen (Fig. 2), the line of section passed through the centre of the *os calcis* posteriorly, and between the second and third toes anteriorly, passing between the metatarsal

B

bones of these toes and through the remains of the middle cuneiform and scaphoid bones. On examining

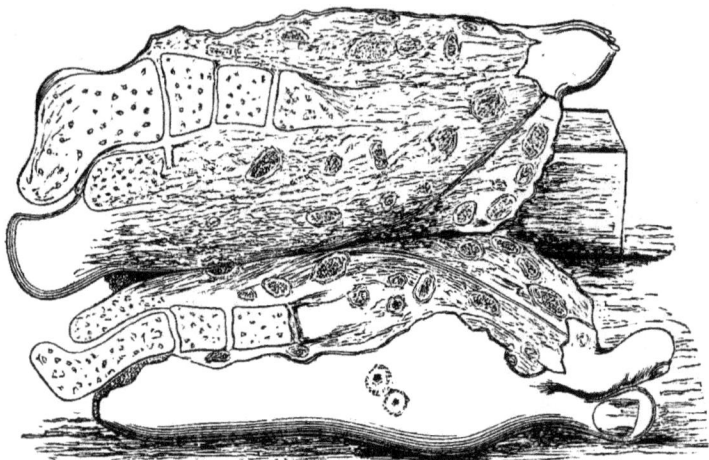

Fig. 2.—Section of a foot affected with the Pale variety of the disease.

the divided surfaces, the foot was seen to be greatly thickened below the line of the bones. The thickening had occurred both below and above the plantar fascia, foci of degeneration being present in both situations, although more abundantly below than above the fascia.

These foci consisted of cavities lined by smooth membrane and containing gelatinous and caseous matter, or distinct roe-like masses of minute rounded parti-cles. These roe-like aggregations were quite free in the cavities, and were surrounded with more or less mucoid or gelatinoid semi-fluid material. In some instances the cavities appeared to have penetrated the plantar fascia, or rather, perhaps, to have passed be-tween the several strips of its tissue. They presented a curiously symmetrical arrangement in some places, especially immediately beneath the skin, where the normal series of fat masses was in great part replaced by a row of cavities containing roe-like bodies. These cavities in many cases coincided in size and form with

Cavities in the tis-sues: their nature and contents.

the loculi usually occupied by fat—their lining membrane, although somewhat thicker, being composed of the same anatomical elements as those normally separating and limiting the masses of fat, and only differing from the normal partitions in being denser and containing a somewhat larger proportion of common connective tissue in relation to the elastic fibres. In some cases the cavities were perfectly isolated, occurring among healthy fat-masses, in others they were close to one another, only separated by their limiting membranes; in others they communicated directly or indirectly with one another, and in some cases two or more appeared to have coalesced entirely, so as to form one large, frequently somewhat irregular, cavity. In almost all instances the openings on the surface of the foot were found to lead by means of channels into such cavities, whilst another series of channels connected cavities or sets of cavities with one another. Similar cavities containing degenerate material were also present in the subcutaneous fat of the dorsal aspect of the foot.

The bones, although softened and oily in texture, were in great part distinctly traceable, especially towards the inner half of the foot, but even here the base of the second metatarsal bone was disorganised and completely obscured by the degeneration. The muscular and tendinous structures were little, if at all, affected, and appeared to have contributed to the deformity of the foot by their action on the soft and weakened bones, although the greater part of the extreme flattening of the foot was, no doubt, due to the extent of the disease in the fat and connective tissue.

Condition of the bones.

The membranous lining of the cavities and the various materials contained in the latter were carefully examined microscopically. The caseous matter and roe-like masses were found to consist of oily matter in various conditions. The caseous matter was formed of yellowish amorphous material mingled with oil globules; it was readily acted

Microscopic examinations.

on by liquor potassæ, and when treated with this re-
agent frequently gave rise to an abundance of tubes,
filaments, and globules of myeline. The particles forming the roe-like masses were composed of a large central
mass or nucleus of similar caseous matter densely
clothed with radiating crystals. These, when the particles
were compressed beneath a cover-glass, appeared as
fringes of a feathery aspect surrounding a central mass
of amorphous matter, and when a
current was induced by the addition
of a drop of water to the slide, the
crystalline fringes were seen to become bent in the direction of the
current, as may be observed in the
adjoining woodcut—Fig. 3. Prolonged and careful microscopic examination failed to reveal the presence
of any fungoid elements notwithstanding the use of most various re-
agents. Some of the particles having
been first treated with chloroform
were immersed in liquor potassæ
and kept under observation during
several weeks. They appeared at

Fig. 3.—A roe-like
particle under a moderate
power, with feathery
crystals adherent to it;
the latter curved at one
part owing to a current
being induced on the
slide. × 100.

first to be partially dissolved, and were subsequently
deposited in the form of a whitish gelatinous layer
on the side of the test tube in which they were kept.
The material of this layer was found to consist almost
entirely of beautiful tubes, filaments, and cysts of myeline
of every conceivable form, affording an excellent opportunity for the study of the many curious and complex
forms which matter of such nature is capable of
assuming (vide Fig. 4, page 34.)

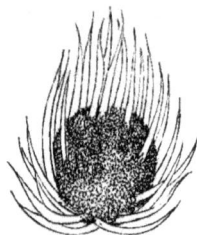

SPECIMEN III.—A foot and ankle-joint (Plate I,

Description of Spe-
cimen III—Roe-like
bodies and chalky
crystalline masses.

Fig 1.) This foot was enormously
enlarged transversely, and the toes
were shortened, turned upwards, and
more or less drawn backwards into the foot, so that
the latter presented a peculiarly thick, 'stumpy' aspect.

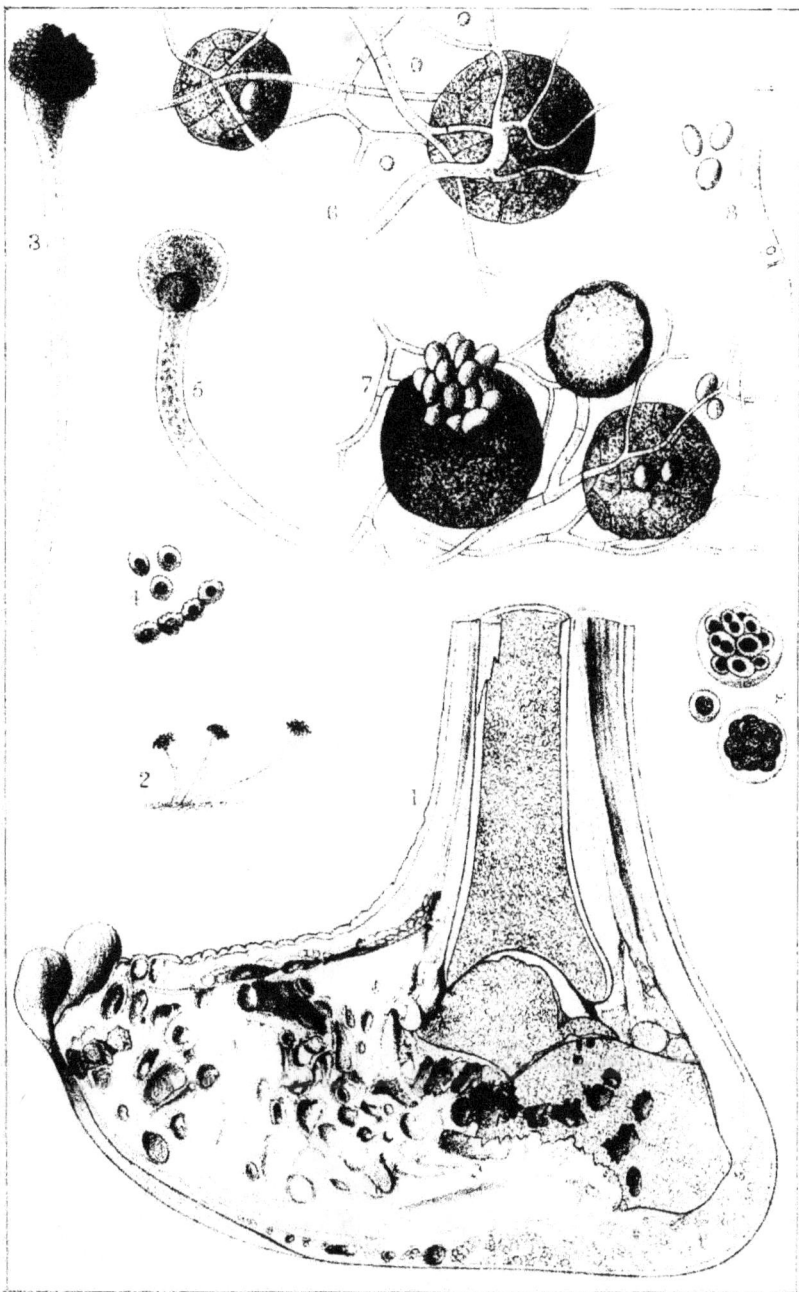

Plate I.

THE FUNGUS - DISEASE OF INDIA

PALE VARIETY &c.

Lithographed in Colors at the Surveyor General's Office, Calcutta October 1875.

The shortening and upturning of the toes were specially marked in the case of the second one, where the distortion had proceeded so far that the tip of the toe projected upwards on the dorsum of the foot; the nail resting on the dorsal surface of the foot and only becoming visible when the toe was forcibly bent forwards in some degree. On both dorsal and plantar aspects of the foot, there were numerous mammillated projections surrounding orifices of the diameter of crow or goose-quills, which communicated with channels penetrating the substance of the foot, and from which soft granular matter could be forced by pressure. Amputation had been performed through the lower fourth of the leg.

A section was carried completely through the foot, dividing the tissues from the space between the second and third toes to the centre of the calcaneum and thence upwards through the astragalus and middle of the tibia. The entire section was performed with a knife from an ordinary dissecting case, which passed through the bones with the greatest ease save towards the upper portion of the tibia, where a certain amount of resistance was

---

EXPLANATION OF PLATE I.

1. Section of a foot affected with the Pale variety of the disease, showing cavities and channels in the substance of the tissues. Isolated masses of subcutaneous fat of the sole of the foot are seen to be affected by the degeneration (*vide* page 20.)
2. Rose-colored variety of *Aspergillus* developed on the roe-like masses of the degeneration (*vide* page 77.) × 60.
3. Separate filament of the *Aspergillus* more highly magnified, showing the staining of the plasma. × 250.
4. Spores of *Aspergillus* from the same cultivation, showing normal and rose-colored varieties. × 950.
5. Young head of *Mucor* from the same cultivation, showing red-coloring of the contents. × 250.
6. *Eurotium* developed on the surface of a fluid in which portions of the degenerate material from a foot affected with the pale variety of the disease, were immersed (*vide* page 72.) × 400.
7. Rose-colored variety of the same *Eurotium* occurring beneath the fluid in the same cultivation. × 400.
8. Specimens of spores and a portion of a filament from *Eurotium* developed on cartilage in Calcutta. × 600.
9. Rose-colored cells (*Algæ?*) developed in a cultivation of choleraic excreta in water. × 300.

experienced and where the bone presented an apparently normal aspect. The disease of the tarsal bones was extremely advanced.

Condition of the bones.

The astragalus retained its normal outline, but was extremely open in texture internally, the spaces in the bony tissue being full of yellow oily matter, and here and there containing distinct aggregations of roe-like particles. The greater portion of the front half of the os calcis was reduced to a soft pulp containing irregular excavations bathed in oily fluid and abounding in roe-like particles. The posterior half resembled the astragalus in condition generally, but contained several distinct cavities of considerable size containing roe-like bodies. The remainder of the tarsal bones in the line of section were almost entirely reduced to a softened, undifferentiated mass, riddled with irregular cavities, and in which mere fragments of bone remained distinguishable, the arch of the foot being entirely obliterated, and even the faintest indications of the individual bones having been destroyed. The bases of the first phalanges of the toes were the first recognisable osseous elements anteriorly, and even these were extremely softened, opened out, and oily in texture. Considering the extreme degree of the degeneration, it was curious to observe how little the muscular tissue was affected, the fibres being apparently unaltered, and presenting well marked striæ in almost all the fragments which were subjected to microscopic examination.

The fatty tissue throughout the entire foot was, however, very much altered and degenerated. The subcutaneous fat showed various stages of degeneration with great distinctness, the nests of fat-cells appearing in three distinct forms: (a) The normal loculi of connective tissue filled with apparently healthy fat, the capsule containing the fat being seemingly unaltered, and the cells of the latter not being readily separable from it. This condition was specially present towards the posterior portion of the sole and behind the heel. (b) Loculi which presented pretty much the same appearances as

Various stages of degeneration among the fatty tissues.

those in the previous form, but in which the contents
were more or less gelatinous, caseous, or waxy in appearance and consistence ; in many cases, in fact, approaching more or less closely in their characters to those
presented by the ceruminous secretions of the ear. Two
or more loculi were here and there blended to a greater
or less extent, or were almost united into a common
cavity of larger size. The fatty contents were easily
removed, leaving cavities closely resembling those presently to be described, and only differing from them in
the less consistent nature of their lining membranes.
(c) The cavities here were enlarged, or rather the septa
between the normal loculi were more or less completely
absorbed or thrust aside, in some cases having been
entirely obliterated, and in others persisting in a more
or less fragmentary condition as threads or pillars of
connective tissue. These cavities were occupied by
masses of circular, yellowish-white grains or particles,
like small seeds or ova, aggregated into masses of various sizes, and evidently forming the roe-like bodies so
constantly described as characteristic of the discharges
and tissues in this variety of the Madura disease.

The cavities in the deeper tissues of the foot were
exactly similar in appearance to those
occupying the subcutaneous fat, and,
likethem, contained oily and fatty matter in various forms,
but principally in that of roe-like masses. Many of the
cavities, both superficial and deep, were quite isolated and
unconnected with any others, or with the surface, whilst
others communicated freely with one another either
directly, or by means of channels, and some of the more
superficial also communicated with the exterior in a
similar fashion. In the latter case, the channels connected with the cavities opened on the mammillations
previously mentioned as occurring on the integument
of the foot. The lining membrane of the channels and
cavities—whether occupying the subcutaneous or interstitial adipose tissue, or the sites of disintegrated bone—
was throughout the same ; and on microscopic examination was found to consist of connective tissue abounding more or less in elastic fibres.

The various modifications of fatty matter above
described could be seen to merge into one another by
insensible degrees throughout the preparation. In some
loculi individual lobules of fat had passed more or less
completely into the ceruminous condition, whilst the
remaining ones were to all appearance perfectly normal,

Transitions between
normal fat and dege-
nerate products.
and in those cavities in which all
normal fat had disappeared, the con-
tents shaded off gradually from yellowish, ceruminous,
amorphous masses through a series of intermediate forms
into the characteristic roe-like particles. Apparently a
still further stage of the degeneration was represented
by specimens of the latter, which, in place of their
normal yellowish colour and waxy consistence, presented
a glistening white colour and friable texture, and resembled, when in mass, small lumps of chalk. It will be
seen that, in so far as the unaided senses were concerned, no hard-and-fast line could be drawn between the
normal fat of the tissues at one end of the series of
modified forms, and the thoroughly degenerate chalky
masses at the other, for an almost infinite series of intermediate steps was present. The same remark also holds
good of the results of careful microscopic examinations
also. Starting with normal masses of fat, the series
could be traced through gradual stages in which the
contents of the cells became more or less completely
condensed into waxy amorphous masses, whilst the cell
walls became more and more obscured until a uniform
mass of the former, still retaining a somewhat cellular
arrangement, was all that remained. From this the
series proceeded through a set of forms characterised by
increasing condensation of the material and the appearance of feathery crystals on the surface, passing on into
the characteristic fringed roe-like particles (Fig. 3, p. 20),
and culminating in the chalky masses of acicular
crystals.

All the varieties of morbid material present in this

Results of micros-
copic examination.
case were carefully ransacked with
the aid of the most various re-agents
and appliances, with the view of ascertaining the presence of any vegetable organisms or other foreign bodies

as constituents of them, but entirely in vain. It was
quite clear that in this case, at all events, we had merely
to deal with a degeneration of the normal constituents
of the tissues, unassociated with, and uncomplicated by,
the presence of any extraneous elements.

SPECIMEN IV.—This consisted of a portion of skin
and subcutaneous tissue from the sole of the foot in a
case where the diseased condition was limited to the
textures between the plantar fascia and the integument
of the sole of the foot.

There were numerous slight elevations on the surface
of the skin, beneath which minute dark coloured points
could be seen. These were hard to the touch, and
in some cases small openings could be detected
Description of Speci-
menIV—Early stage of
the disease. leading inwards towards them from
the surface. On dissecting down
upon them, these points were found to consist of isolated dull, yellowish, more or less spherical bodies of firm,
waxy consistence (*vide* Plate II, Fig. 5). They were
easily compressible, and spread out into a greasy smear
on the surface of the glass on which they were examined. Both as regards microscopical appearance and
effects of re-agents they coincided exactly with the ceruminous masses of the previous specimen (page 25), or
with the nuclei of the common roe-like particles. The
subcutaneous fat was carefully examined under a low
magnifying power, and a sprinkling of similar bodies
was detected in and removed from it. It was quite
evident that these were local degenerations of portions
of the normal fatty tissue, lobules or aggregations of fat
cells being discovered in various stages of modification
from mere slight condensation of the contents of the cells
up to the formation of firm, waxy grains or concretions,
which, in the more advanced cases, had lost all organic
connection with the surrounding tissues, and were ma-
nifestly only capable of acting as foreign bodies (Plate
II, Figs. 5-6).

Microscopic examinations here, too, failed to show
any traces of the presence of vegetable organisms, the

degenerated material consisting solely of waxy, amorphous matter. No distinct roe-like particles were to be found by the unaided senses, and the microscope showed an entire absence of fringes or other crystalline forms in connection with the concretions. In this case the degeneration was evidently merely commencing, and *Commencing degeneration.* had not yet advanced so far as to pass on to the formation of crystals, but as the case was one of comparatively short duration —the patient had only suffered from the disease for one year—this was only what might, perhaps, have been expected, and the probability is that the absence of the characteristic roe-like particles was due to this, and not to any peculiarity in the morbid process.

SPECIMEN V.—A collection of the roe-like particles discharged from the foot in a case previous to amputation.

These presented no special peculiarities, and were *Description of Specimen V—Roe-like particles.* composed of the usual aggregations of masses of fatty matter of waxy consistence fringed with feathery crystals. No signs of fungal or other vegetable elements could be detected in them.

SPECIMEN VI.—A specimen of diseased tissues from *Description of Specimen VI—Sundried.* a foot, comprising both bones and soft parts, which had been dried in the sun. This was obtained in order to provide materials for cultivation, and presented nothing in any way peculiar. It contained an abundance of the characteristic roe-like bodies, and, as usual, was devoid of all fungal elements.

SPECIMEN VII.—This consisted of transverse sections through the lower portion of the leg in a case of this form of the disease.

All the fatty and fibrous tissues were extremely gela-*Description of Specimen VII—Red particles.* tinous, and the preparations were characterised by an extreme profusion of minute, bright rose-coloured bodies, which were sprinkled over the surface of the tissues and formed an abundant deposit at the bottom of the fluid in which the specimen was preserved. They were so abundant as to give the sections the appearance of having been sprinkled with red pepper, and at once to attract attention to their presence even whilst still in the bottle in which they were preserved. On careful examination they appeared to be mainly, if not wholly, confined to the surfaces of the sections, as in no instance could it be clearly ascertained that they were present in freshly exposed portions of the tissues. As a rule, they appeared to be quite loose in the softened gelatinous matter of the degenerated tissues, but here and there they seemed to be entangled amongst, or attached to filaments of, connective tissue. Their intimate nature will be described farther on, but it may in the meantime be stated that they showed no signs of containing any fungal elements, or of being in any way related to such bodies ; and that we are strongly inclined to believe that the number of them present in the specimen increased whilst it remained in our hands.

CHAPTER IV.

HAVING now given some examples of the materials illustrative of this form of the disease which we have examined, and which have formed the basis for our views regarding its nature and causation, we may next proceed briefly to state what these views are. We shall confine our attention at present to it and leave the question of its relation to the other variety to be discussed at a subsequent page. We have, as the above illustrative cases may serve to show, totally and absolutely failed to identify the presence of any fungal or other parasitic elements in any of the specimens which we have examined, and we believe that we have good grounds for denying the necessary coincidence, and consequently, much more the causative connection of the presence of any parasitic organisms at all with the morbid changes present.

The degeneration may occur without the local presence of any parasitic organisms.

We have studied very various stages of the disease, and in all alike has there been an absence of any demonstrable parasites; but more than this, we have been able to trace out a series of modifications of the elements of the normal tissues terminating in lesions and degenerations which are quite capable of accounting for all the appearances present in the most advanced stages, and which, therefore, render the assumption of the essential agency of a parasite not merely unnecessary, but even inadmissible. Why this degeneration should occur, and why it should be specially localised in the extremities, we cannot say, but we believe that we have good grounds for the assertion that this variety of the disease primarily is essentially a degeneration of the fatty tissues independent of the local presence or influence of any parasites whatever.

In a very early stage of the disease, as, for instance, in Specimen IV (page 27), we found mere alterations in the normal fat,

The disease essentially a degeneration of the fatty tissues.

and in more advanced cases we have been able to trace such degenerative changes onwards. That the degeneration is essentially one of the fatty tissues, is not only evident from the nature of its ultimate products, but from the localisation of the primary foci of the diseased action. These foci are invariably situated in localities abounding in fat, in the sub-cutaneous adipose tissue, in the sub-fascial or inter-muscular connective tissue, and in the cancellated tissue of bones, and specially in spongy bones abounding in fatty matter.

The degenerative process appears to consist in a gradual condensation and inspissation of the contents of the fat cells, with

Nature of the degenerative process.

a coincident diminution and disappearance of the vascular supply of the lobes and lobules of the adipose tissue, and an ultimate solution of the interstitial connective tissue and cell membranes. The latter process appears to occur by mucoid or gelatinoid softening, and to result in the formation of the gelatinous matter in which the altered constituents of the fat are so frequently found to be embedded. Whether the affection, however, primarily originates in the fat itself, the connective tissue, or the lymph-spaces, we are not in a position to state. Once such a degenerative process has occurred, the masses of fatty concretions and gelatinous substance resulting from it are virtually portions of dead matter, really external to, and unconnected with, the economy, and little prone to change save in so far as the fatty constituents tend towards the assumption of crystalline forms. Such foreign extraneous substances must naturally tend to excite a certain amount of irritation in the surrounding tissues, causing a thickening of the connective tissues around them, and the gradual formation of cyst-like cavities so characteristic of the disease.

A further progress of the irritant action may ultimately lead these cysts to open into one another, thereby forming irregular cavities, and cause the formation of channels lined with a membrane of connective tissue, and in many cases opening externally and allowing of the escape of the products of the degeneration.

The degree to which the degeneration may proceed varies greatly in different instances, as also does the proportion which the fatty and gelatinous products bear to one another.

The proportion of gelatinoid and fatty products differ in various specimens.

In some cases we find roe-like masses and other crystalline elements in comparatively small proportion, while the tissues are bathed in an abundance of oleo-gelatinous fluid. In other instances the separation of the fatty and gelatinoid materials is found to have advanced to a high degree, and distinct cavities containing roe-like masses of fatty concretions characterise the tissues. Once, however, the gelatinoid degeneration of the connective tissues and an alteration in the fat cells with obliteration of the vascular supply have occurred, it is not necessary that distinct concretions should form in order to cause the degenerate matter to act as a foreign body and lead to the formation of cavities, with channels and openings for its discharge. Specimen I (page 15) afforded a characteristic example of this; for in it, although the degeneration was widely diffused and the characteristic openings were present on the surface, the amount of roe-like, crystalline concretions was comparatively small.

The amount and nature of deformity present in different instances vary with the degree in which the various tissues have been involved, and in which an hypertrophy of the fat and connective tissues has coincided with the degeneration.

Characters and causes of deformities present in different instances.

In almost all cases there is an apparent thickening of the affected extremities, which is sometimes real and due to thickening of the masses of connective tissue in some places, and to their being opened out into cavities in others. An apparent thickening may, however, be to a great extent independent of any hypertrophic changes, being in many cases due to a folding or crushing together of the tissues induced by the action of the muscles and tendons on the softened non-resistent bones. In the case of the lower extremity, the mere mechanical weight of the body in many cases contributes to the production of deformity, as may frequently be seen in cases where the calcaneum has been much affected by the degeneration. The precise nature of the deformity is, of course, determined by the degree in which all these factors come into play ; but one of the most common results of their action on the lower extremity (in which the disease most frequently occurs) is an obliteration of the arch of the foot and a turning upwards, or even backwards, of the toes. The latter phenomenon is due to muscular action, and may cause it to appear as though a great amount of thickening of the tissues of the sole had occurred, when, in fact, little or nothing of the kind has taken place.

In describing the specimens, reference has been already made to the characters of the various morbid products constituting the ultimate results of the degeneration, and this may suffice in so far as the majority of them are concerned. There are, however, one or two points regarding which somewhat fuller details appear to be necessary. These refer to the ordinary fatty concretions, and specially to the character and nature of the peculiar coloured particles which occurred in such abundance in Specimen VII (page 28).

Special description of certain morbid products.

In so far as the common fatty concretions are concerned, it is rather a caution as to the interpretation of phenomena connected with them than any further description which we wish to give here. As previously mentioned, these concretions, under the influence of various re-agents, very readily give origin to an abundance of that curious and ill-defined substance which Virchow has termed myeline. A development of myeline is specially prone

Myeline.

to occur where portions of the fatty matter, roe-like masses, &c., freshly removed from an alcoholic preparation, are subjected to the action of liquor potassæ. The multifarious and highly complex forms of tubes, filaments, globules, and cysts, which may frequently be observed to become developed—shooting out, and, as it were, growing from the globules and aggregations of fatty matter, are wonderful, and such that they could hardly be believed to owe their origin to any such process or material were not their development distinctly traceable through all its stages.

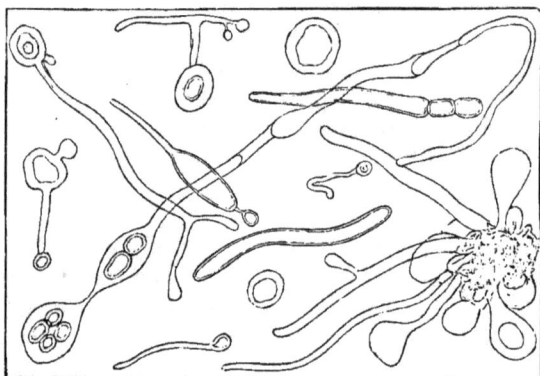

Fig. 4.—Various fungi-like forms assumed by 'Myeline' × 500.

From the extremely organised nature of their appearance, they are, as the accompanying figure will show, peculiarly liable to be mistaken for fungal growths, especially by those who are unused to the practical study of such bodies and to the various appearances presented by complex oily compounds, and it is necessary that very great caution should be exercised in the interpretation of such phenomena. Bodies of this nature are usually very transitory, but they may persist for weeks, as was exemplified in the preparation referred to in the description of Specimen II (page 20), and they may in some cases be even suffered to dry up more or less completely without losing their peculiar forms.

The physical conditions, moulding a plastic semi-fluid material into peculiar forms, probably produce much the Often difficult to distinguish vitalised from non-vitalised products. same effects, whether the material acted upon be endowed with vitality or not, so that the close resemblance of these organic to truly organised forms need be no special cause for surprise. We have, however, in the course of investigation been more and more strongly impressed with the necessity of caution in deciding on the nature of equivocal bodies merely from their outward appearance and morphological characters, and we believe that this necessity is one which holds good, not only in regard to the morbid products of the disease forming the subject of the present report, but also with equal force to the interpretation of the appearances present in many other cases, and specially in the so-called parasitic skin diseases.

CHAPTER V.

THE peculiar red particles referred to as being pre-
Red particles.   sent in Specimen VII (page 28) de-
mand more special consideration. As previously mentioned, on consulting the literature of the subject, it will
be found that they are of such rare occurrence in connection with the disease, that they can hardly be regarded as characteristic of it. Considerable weight has,
however, been laid on their occasional presence, in
favour of the fungal or parasitic nature of the degeneration, and we therefore gladly availed ourselves of
the excellent opportunities which we had of closely
investigating their nature.

In the present case, the red coloring was absolutely
confined to the particles; there was no staining of the
tissues in connection with which they occurred. The
particles, as previously stated, immediately attracted
attention, as an abundant sprinkling of minute, bright,
red points or grains scattered over the tissues and deposited on the sides and bottom of the vessel containing
the preparation. Their size varied considerably in different instances, but in the greater number ranged from
$\frac{1}{120}'' \times \frac{1}{170}''$ to $\frac{1}{90}'' \times \frac{1}{120}''$. Their outline was generally rounded or oval, but many more or less irregular
forms also occurred; these might, however, be almost
always ascribed to the occurrence of fracture or rupture
of the commoner forms, or to the union of several particles into an aggregate (*vide* Plate II, Figs. 3—4).

The figures in the plate show the principal varieties
of forms present, and that they were all modifications of
the round or oval primary one. Many of them, in place
of having an even surface, were more or less tubercu-

lated or knotted; others were constricted in the middle, or even actually separated into two portions with an intervening space; others were aggregated longitudinally in a moniliform fashion, or formed irregular heaps; whilst others, again, were ruptured and, as it were, unfolded. The colour, when fully developed, appeared bright vermilion to the naked eye, and under the microscope passed from this into a rosy carmine, according to the degree of magnifying power employed. The colour of the particles was, however, by no means uniform in intensity in all instances, a faint red or pinkish tinge being all that could be determined in many, whilst in others the red colouring was entirely absent, and they were of a dull buff or yellowish hue. The latter particles did not, in other respects, in any way differ from the most highly colored particles in appearance. In some cases, as fractured specimens showed, the particles were solid and seemingly homogeneous throughout, but in others they appeared to contain a central cavity—an appearance which, as will appear farther on, was not a deceptive one.

When examined under comparatively high powers, from 400 to 1,500 diameters linear, Their microscopic structure. they appeared to be composed of a finely molecular material. In some instances they presented a homogeneous aspect, but in others they had more or less of a cellular appearance, being marked out into areas by obscure double lines. This appearance was, in some cases, not dependent on any true cellular structure, but was due to the existence of irregular fissures running through the substance of the particle and extending from the central cavity when the latter was present. In other instances, however, the phenomenon appeared to be of a different nature, and the structure of the particles seemed yet to retain the traces of the fat cells out of which they had been formed.

Beyond these characters nothing could be ascertained regarding the nature of these particles Behaviour with various re-agents. by microscopic examination alone, and recourse was accordingly had to the use of re-agents. In working at the chemistry of the subject, we had the great benefit of the advice of an accomplished chemist, Mr. C. H. Wood, the Quinologist to Government, who not only suggested the use of various tests, but also tried some of them for us himself. We shall now give an account of the effects produced by the various methods and re-agents employed, and shall subsequently state the conclusions at which we have arrived in regard to the nature of these curious bodies. It was very easy to procure large numbers of the particles free from other materials, as, owing to the fact that their specific gravity is very high, they were rapidly deposited when shaken up with water and allowed to subside.

1. *Liquor Potassæ.*—This at once changed the rosy color to a dull buff-yellow, but produced no further effect when the ordinary pharmacopocial preparation was used; even when the particles remained for prolonged periods immersed in an excess of the re-agent. When, however, a concentrated solution was resorted to, the particles were slowly dissolved.

2. *Liquor Ammoniæ.*—The effects produced by this re-agent were precisely similar to those of the dilute liquor potassæ.

3. *Hydrochloric Acid.*—This when dilute produced no effect, save somewhat brightening the red colour in some instances. When applied to specimens which had been previously treated with potash or ammonia, the red coloring was in general at once restored, and the processes of discharge and restoration of colour could be frequently repeated by means of alternate applications of the alkaline and acid re-agents.

4. *Nitric Acid.*—The effects of this when dilute were precisely similar to those of the previous re-agent.

5. *Sulphuric Acid.*—This when weak acted similarly to the other acids. When strong, it broke up and partially dissolved the particles.

6. *Acetic Acid.*—The action of this was precisely similar to that of the weak mineral acids.

7. *Chromic Acid.*—This at once destroyed the colouring of the particles on coming in contact with them. A

development of bubbles of gas then, generally, occurred within the substance of the particles, more especially in those containing a distinct cavity in their interior, and the formation of such bubbles, followed by their gradual expulsion through fissures, where such were present, continued for some time. Short tubes and globules resembling myeline were then gradually given off from the surface of the particle, and, growing outwards, ultimately were detached from it. After this the mass became more and more obscure and dimly molecular, and finally remained as an indistinct molecular flake.

8. *Liquor Iodi.*—This produced no effect, save somewhat browning the bright rosy tint of the particles where it came into contact with them.

9. *Benzene.*—Some particles having been carefully prepared by successive washings with water, alcohol and ether were then subjected to the action of boiling benzene for more than half an hour. Their colour, which had been partially discharged by the action of the alcohol and ether, entirely disappeared and they assumed a somewhat fatty aspect. They were, however, otherwise unaltered and showed no tendency towards solution.

11. *Chloroform.*—This produced much the same effects as benzene.

12. *Sulphide of Carbon.*—The action of this resembled that of the two previous re-agents.

13. *Heated Oil.*—Prolonged immersion in olive oil at 212° F. produced no effect on the particles, save, perhaps, a slight alteration in their colour.

14. *Heat.*—On placing particles on a capsule or sheet of platinum and exposing them cautiously to the heat of a spirit lamp, they were found to become blackened almost immediately, their surfaces assuming a jet black color and glistening appearance, as though they were partially melted.

Effects of heat on the red particles.

At the same time their outline frequently became somewhat irregular, and a distinct but very transitory smell resembling that of burned feathers was given off. On subsequently applying the blow-pipe and subjecting them to a bright red heat for a moment, the particles were found on examination to have become partially white—in many cases almost entirely so—a mere sprinkling of minute black points remaining on the surface. When still further heated, all blackness finally disappeared, and the particles were either pure white, or partially white and partially rusty brown, in colour. Though possibly somewhat smaller than they had been previous to exposure to heat, they yet retained their characteristic forms almost intact, and by careful manipulation could be removed entire and submitted to microscopic examination. They were then found to consist of shells or skeletons of inorganic matter, the particles of which had a more or less crystalline aspect.

Their outlines, and general forms under the microscope, too, were very frequently almost identical with those of the original red particles. The material of which they were composed was either entirely colourless, or more or less stained, of a bright rusty-brown or yellowish tint. When the former was the case, they were entirely soluble in weak acids, the solution varying in rapidity in different instances. In some cases it was accomplished quietly and without any evolution of gas, whilst in others effervescence occurred in various degrees. When, however, any rusty-brown matter was present, this remained in great part unaffected by dilute acids, but was readily soluble in strong hydrochloric acid, and if ferrocyanide of potassium were then added to the solution, an immediate development of blue colour took place. The presence of considerable quantities of iron in the ash of the particles may, perhaps, be even more strikingly demonstrated, in many instances, by treating the skeletons of the particles with weak acid whilst still on the platinum, and then adding the ferrocyanide, when each particle immediately becomes of a deep Prussian blue.

Such have been the result of our investigations into the structure and composition of these peculiar bodies, and we have now to consider the question of their real nature. Save in regard to some vague points of form, they present

Nature of these bodies.

nothing which can in any way suggest that they are of a vegetable or parasitic nature. Even in regard to form, too, they show nothing which may not frequently be found in concretions of various kinds ; for, although some of the appearances may in some degree appear to suggest a process of multiplication by cell division, they may all be readily accounted for by mere mechanical processes of aggregation and fracture. Taking everything into consideration, we have no hesitation in affirming them to be mere concretions, containing varying proportions of mineral matter in the form of phosphates and carbonates, and, in many cases, combined with a considerable quantity of iron. The presence of carbonates, phosphates, and of iron, was clearly demonstrated by the action of re-agents.

To what their brilliant rosy coloration is due, we are

Cause of their colour uncertain.

unable satisfactorily to determine ; but, as we shall hereafter see, the fatty matter of the degenerate tissues in the pale variety of the Madura disease has, under certain circumstances, a tendency to give rise to the development of such colouring. The red colouring is, moreover, not an essential character in the concretions ; for, as previously mentioned, numerous specimens occurred of precisely similar nature to the most highly coloured ones, save in being of a buff or yellowish hue in place of bright carmine, whilst many other intermediate forms were present showing various degrees of staining. The specimen in which they occurred was preserved in strong glycerine, and there appeared to be a gradual but considerable increase in their numbers whilst it was kept under observation. In studying the conditions under which a development of red colouring matter occurs in connection with the fatty products of the ochroid variety of the Madura disease, we have observed that one of them appears to be the existence of more or less decided acidity, and it is noteworthy that, in the present instance, the glycerine was distinctly acid in re-action. The results of attempts at cultivation of the red particles will be

given subsequently, but in the meantime we would repeat
that they appear to us to be mere concretions, probably
formed from the degenerated tissues—the proportion of
constituents furnished by the latter varying in different
instances. Possibly they owe their red hue to a substance analogous to the colouring matter of the blood—
just as other pigmentary substances are believed to do.

CHAPTER VI.

A DESCRIPTION OF SPECIMENS ILLUSTRATIVE OF THE DARK VARIETY
OF THE FUNGUS-DISEASE OF INDIA.

HAVING given a minute description of several ex-

Illustrative speci-
mens of the dark vari-
ety.

amples of the pale variety of the
fungus-disease, we now proceed to give
a similar description of a few typical specimens of the
dark variety. Instead, however, of giving a full account
of the peculiar substance which is characteristic of all of
them, we shall defer the details of the more minute
investigations of it until the general appearance of the
specimens has been described. This will economise space
without sacrificing exactness, for this dark substance
does not materially vary in the different specimens.

SPECIMEN I.—A glance at the accompanying sketch

Specimen I—Section
of a foot.

of a longitudinal section of the left
foot of a native will convey a more
accurate conception of the state of the tissues in this
disease than any verbal description. An ordinary scalpel
was made to pass through the tissues from the inter-
digital space between the second and third toe in a line
towards the middle of the tibia and through the centre
of the ankle joint. The scalpel passed readily through
all the tissues, except the tibia and the portion of the
astragalus articulating with it. The foot is enlarged
in all directions; the toes are turned upwards in the same
manner as may be observed in the Specimen in Plate I,
delineating the pale variety; and there are several openings on the surface which may generally be found to
be continuous with a cavity in the tissue below. Some
of the orifices are plugged, more or less completely, by
irregular-shaped little aggregations of black substance
which can be picked out. On examining the section,
the outlines of the tarsal bones cannot be made out;
but, as the figure shows, the bones occupy an irregular

space, perforated by numerous excavations in all directions. The middle portion of the metatarsal bone, ex-

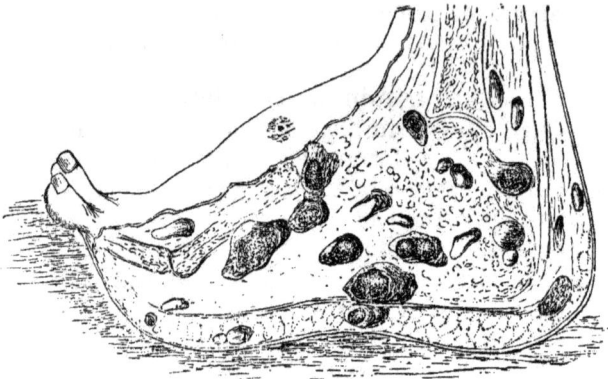

Fig. 5.—A section through an affected foot showing numerous cavities
with dark masses *in situ.* Isolated areas of affected tissue in the subcutaneous
fat of the sole are also distinguishable.

posed by the section, is found to be broken down, and
the arch of the foot completely given way, so that the
natural direction of the longer bones of the foot and
the toes has become altered. Between the first phalanx
of the second toe and its corresponding metatarsal bone,
a new articulating surface has been formed on the dorsal
surface of the latter.

The cavities are in some cases isolated, but in others
they communicate by means of one
or more channels with adjoining cav-
ities, the cavities and channels being every where lined
by a more or less dense, smooth membrane of tough
fibrous tissue. The cavities are of very unequal size ; they
vary from being just large enough to contain a pellet of
small-shot to being sufficiently capacious to hold a bullet
with ease. They almost invariably contain irregular
lumps of a dark granular substance, which, more or less
completely, fills the cavities and the channels continuous
with them. Frequently, however, the dark material oc-

Character of the cav-
ities.

cupies but a very small portion of the cavity, even though the cavity be completely isolated. The fatty padding of the sole of the foot appears to be normal, but in two or three places small groups of the lobules have been replaced by cavities containing the dark material.

Numerous fragments of tissues immediately adjoining the cavities were subjected to careful microscopic examination, with results as follow :—

(1.) Muscular tissue from various parts of the foot: Microscopical characters of the ordinary tissues—Muscles. for the most part in a tolerably normal condition; at one spot only could distinctly disintegrated fibres be distinguished. All the samples were subjected to the influence of various re-agents, including the free use of liquor potassæ, but nothing peculiar could be distinguished.

(2.) The membranous lining of the cavities and channels or sinuses. This consists of Fibrous tissues. ordinary fibrous tissue, and is microscopically in no way to be distinguished from similar tissue lining cavities in other abnormal conditions. Such specimens were purposely obtained with a view of instituting comparisons. Frequently, re-duplications of fibrous tissue formed septa, so as to separate a cavity into partially distinct compartments. Neither could we distinguish any unusual appearance in the tissue forming these septa, although they were necessarily in immediate contact with the dark material in every direction. Every re-agent we could think of was resorted to here also.

(3.) Small fragments of bone from immediately adjoining the excavated parts, forming Bones. in fact the osseous boundary of the cavities, were subjected to the action of potash under the microscope. The granular matter filling up the interstices of the bony tissue was rapidly disposed of, but no new structures were brought to light, although the opened-out condition of the cancellated tissue was highly favorable to accurate inspection.

The nature of the dark material will be considered further on in detail; it will be suffi- The dark material. cient here to state that, after subjecting fragments of it to more or less prolonged action of liquor potassæ, numerous filaments and cellular bodies were brought into view.

SPECIMEN II (Plate II, Fig. 2).—This preparation consisted of the right heel and ankle —amputation having been performed through the lower fourth of the tibia and fibula. The fore part of the foot had been removed. It was in an excellent state of preservation. It had been put up by Dr. Mark Robinson of Madura in brine, and forwarded to us without delay, as a specimen of the affection which, although possessing distinct black granules, was not one in which the tissues are extensively diseased.

Specimen II—A heel and ankle.

Dr. Robinson also favoured us with a note as to the condition of the limb before amputation. His words are :—' Right ankle much enlarged, and on both the inner and outer side numerous sinuses—a slight elevation round each opening. A thin yellowish discharge exuded from these openings : no dead bone to be felt by probing. He was unable to walk on this foot.

Appearance of the limb before amputation.

'After removal of the foot, a cut was made through the soft tissues of the ankle, and it was found that they were infiltrated with a yellowish gelatinous substance;

EXPLANATION OF PLATE II.

1. Section of a specimen of the dark variety of the disease, showing a large mass in the substance of the second metatarsal bone, with cavities and channels containing black masses in the soft tissues. An isolated lobule of subcutaneous fat affected by the degeneration is present beneath the base of the first phalanx of the toe (*vide* page 52).

2. Section of another specimen in which the disease was principally developed around the ankle, showing the freedom of the tendons from degeneration, although surrounded by diseased tissue. In the subcutaneous fat of the dorsum of the foot several isolated spots of degeneration have been exposed by the section (*vide* page 46).

3. Red particles from a specimen of the disease (*vide* pages 29, 36), 40.

4. Similar bodies more highly magnified. × 92.

5 6. Specimens showing transition of the subcutaneous fat into the caseous matter forming the concretions in the pale variety of the disease (*vide* page 27)—slightly magnified.

Plate II.

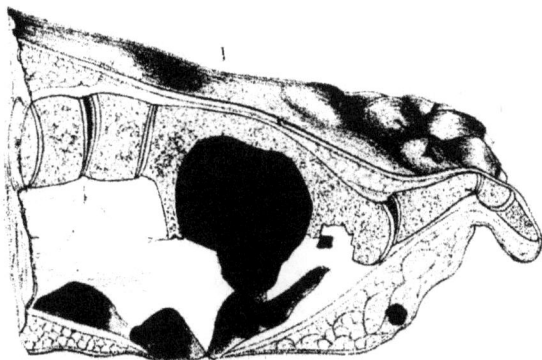

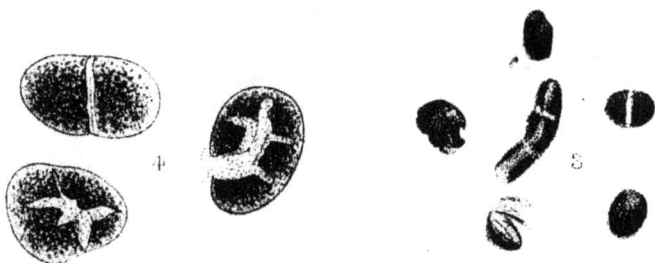

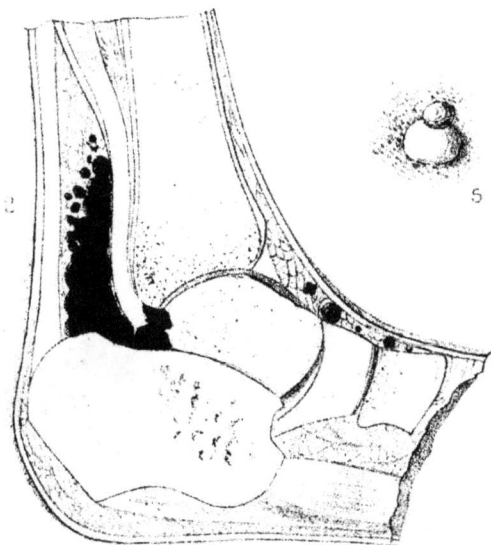

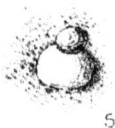

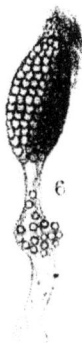

THE FUNGUS-DISEASE OF INDIA

DARK VARIETY &c.

Lithographed in Colors at the Surveyor General's Office, Calcutta October 1875.

the darker patches containing small black granules, the muscular tissue very dark in colour. No section was made through the bones, but they did not appear to be diseased. In the tibio-astragaloid joint there were some flakes of lymph, but the articular surfaces were smooth and bright.'

The lower part of the tibia was softened and the *Appearance of the specimen on section.* cancellated tissue pinkish, especially beneath the cartilage. The shaft was dense, normal in texture, and apparently healthy. The structure of the os calcis and the astragalus was, generally, very dense. The posterior portion of the astragalo-tibial articular surface was excavated and occupied by masses of black substance; there was also a cavity in the anterior part of the os calcis of the size of a small bullet, which was bounded by some very open bone texture. The cartilaginous portion of the os calcis was also eroded and the space occupied by black matter; but the cartilage was not affected to the same extent as the bones, so that projecting portions of it bridged over the hollow occupied by the black matter.

The remaining tarsal bones were softened so as to be cut easily with a scalpel, and in some places the texture was much softened and opened out.

The pad of fat usually found between the tendo Achilles and the posterior surface of the tibia surrounding the deep tendons, was completely converted into a mass of black matter continuous with that in the astragalus and os calcis. The deep tendons, although surrounded by this material, were unaffected and perfectly healthy.

The muscular tissue also was wholly unaffected.

There were various mammillated openings, leading into cavities containing black granules, on the surface of the foot and ankle.

On making sections through the skin of the foot, *Isolated grains of blackened material.* numerous perfectly isolated collections of black granules, like grains of coarse gunpowder, were found to occupy the loculi in the subcutaneous cellular tissue usually occupied by fat. In some an entire lobule of fat appeared to have been converted into a black mass and surrounded by a distinct firm capsule, and in others the lobules were only partially affected—a few black grains, each invested with a capsule, lying among the clusters of cells of the unchanged fatty tissue. This condition will be more minutely described in a subsequent chapter (Chapter VII, page 55).

SPECIMEN III.—A hand amputated about 3 inches above the radio-carpal articulation.
Specimen III—A hand. The cut ends of the two bones of the fore-arm are unaffected. There are several openings on the dorsal surface of the hand, on the front of the wrist,

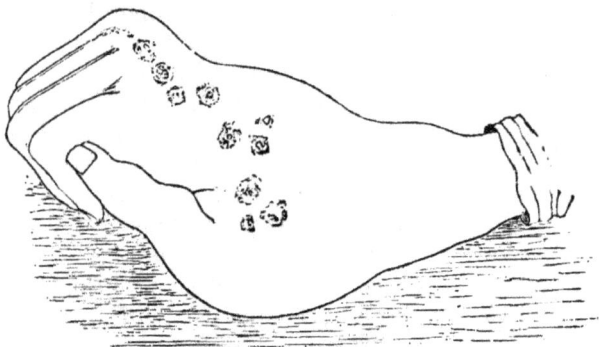

Fig. 6.—Peculiar distortion of the hand in a specimen of the dark variety of the affection.

on the ball of the thumb, and a few along the line of the superficial palmar arch. The hand is swollen and peculiarly distorted, as may be seen from the engraving (Fig. 6). The fingers are not themselves distorted, but are flexed and turned outwards owing to the action of the flexor muscles being continued after the disorganisation of the carpal bones. The nails are unaffected.

A section was made by means of a scalpel in a line extending from the space between the junction of the

second and third phalanx to the point of junction of
the ulna with the radius at the wrist. The knife passed
readily through the os magnum, the semi-lunar bone,
and the outer articular edge of the radius. The distal
end of the os magnum was found to be completely disintegrated, and between it and the upper end of the
second metacarpal bone was lodged a mass of dark-
brown substance, the brown tint predominating towards
the centre, where it might almost be described as presenting a dark-red tint. Several other aggregations of
dark material were found lying between this mass and
the flexor tendons.

In the subcutaneous tissue along the back of the
radius, there were several isolated little cavities, or cysts,
containing aggregations of a cheesy, fatty substance
mixed with black granules. They could be picked out
separately for examination: in the dark masses filaments
could be distinguished after prolonged immersion in
potash; but in the yellowish, roe-like particles, picked
out of the same cavities and similarly treated, no such
filaments could be demonstrated when the particles were
carefully selected. These isolated cavities were limited
to the subcutaneous areolar tissue between the extensor
tendons and the skin of the back of the wrist.

SPECIMEN IV.—Another hand, also amputated a
short distance above the wrist joint.
Specimen IV–A hand. The hand was considerably thickened
and the wrist swollen: the palmar surface was puffed
up, and numerous openings both there, on the dorsal
surface, and between the fingers, communicated with a
large cavity within. A scalpel was carried longitudinally
through the middle of the hand, the bones that still
remained being readily divided, as well as the end of
the radius for a short distance. All the carpal, together
with a great part of the metacarpal bones, were destroyed, the basal half being the portions in the latter most
affected. The phalanges were somewhat softened, but
were not eroded, and contained no black matter. The
metacarpal bone of the third finger was eaten out and

rough, the destruction having proceeded so far as to separate the bone into two rough, irregular fragments. There was not much thickening on the uneroded surfaces. The cavities in the bones were not lined, and the bone presented the appearance of ordinary caries. The cancellous tissue of the end of the radius, and of such portions of the carpal bones as remained, was very porous and widely opened out. Where, however, the cavities were located among the soft tissues, they were lined by a membrane. The tendons were not affected.

The large cavity, referred to as communicating with the surface by means of various channels, occupied the space normal to the carpal bones, and was filled with fragments of these bones mixed with black granular material, which also extended into the channels alongside of the tendons.

The black material, after prolonged immersion in liquor potassæ, was found to contain filaments, but they were by no means so plentiful as ordinarily observed.

Not the slightest indication of any such filaments could be demonstrated in any of the parts, recognisable as tissues, whether diseased or healthy.

SPECIMEN V (Plate II, Fig. 1).—This was a portion of the left foot of a native, which had been removed by Chopart's amputation. There were several openings, with elevated margins, both on the dorsal and plantar surfaces of the foot, out of which dark granules could be picked. There was scarcely any thickening of the tissues of the dorsum.

Specimen V—Anterior portion of the foot.

The preparation was divided longitudinally into four segments. The appearance presented by the first section is delineated at Plate II: the scalpel is seen to have been carried through the middle line of the bones of the second toe. The central portion of the second metatarsal bone was, in great part, occupied by a dark-brown, spherical mass about an inch in diameter, shaped something like a potato and presenting a slightly radiat-

The preparation divided into four segments. Appearance of first section.

ing, finely-striated appearance on section. It was mould-ed to the cavity in which it was lodged, and its projecting nodules fitted accurately into adjoining cavities in the surrounding tissues. The upper portion of the bone was curved, its tissue thickened and hardened, and the lower portion fractured, a splinter being carried in front and behind the dark globular mass, thus aiding in the forma-tion of the cavity. The latter communicated with both the dorsal and plantar surfaces of the foot by means of irregular channels containing small black masses. The middle cuneiform bone was somewhat softened below.

There was another large cavity (visible in this line of section) situated somewhat behind the one just described and above the plantar fascia. It also contained dark tuberculated masses, and opened into several small cavi-ties which communicated with the surface on the sole of the foot. There were other cavities of smaller size.

The second line of section was carried from behind forwards through the middle of the **Appearance of seg-ments in second line of section.** cuboid bone, the base of the fourth metatarsal, and the line between the latter bone and the third metatarsal. In this section the outer boundary of the large cavity was distinguished: it consisted of a delicate fibrous membrane just sufficient to partition off the cavity from another group of cavities and channels. This group appeared to have originated with a cavity in the third metatarsal bone. The base of this bone was intact at its articular surface, and for about a third of an inch forwards, but then became covered with rough, warty nodules of hard bone extending along the entire length of the shaft, the sclerosis being specially marked towards the basal extremity of the bone. Its under and inner surfaces were involved in the large cavity, and were more or less scooped out. Like the second meta-tarsal, this bone was also arched; the phalanx of the third toe was articulated to the dorsal aspect of the cor-responding metatarsal bone; the toe was consequently directed upwards.

The third line of section was carried through the scaphoid, internal cuneiform, and the longer bones of the great toe. There were other centres of disease here also. A similar excavation had taken place in the metatarsal bone of this segment, and the cavity was occupied by a dark globular mass. As in the other bones, the upper surface of this was likewise curved, and the texture extremely dense, and its outer aspect presented a hard nodulated surface. The bones of the phalanges were unaffected. The scaphoid and cuneiform bones were reddish in the centre, as if from blood staining: the colour faded on exposure to air. Nothing peculiar could be detected in the reddish substance when examined under a microscope.

Appearance of segments in third line of section.

The tubercles along the affected metatarsal bones consisted of small, hollow, closed cavities, which could be shaved from the surface of the bone. Some were rounded elevations, like miniature limpet shells ; others were elongated and even tubular. Their osseous walls were thin and very dense, and sometimes projecting spicules of bone were given off from them internally. Their contents consisted mainly of fat with a mixture of fibrous and connective-tissue corpuscles.

Osseous tubercles along the metatarsal bones.

The black material was microscopically identical with the similar substance in other preparations—that is to say, it contained the usual filaments, but none of these could be found in either the muscular, osseous, or fibrous tissues of the surrounding parts, although carefully searched for by every known method.

CHAPTER VII.

PHYSICAL CHARACTERS AND RELATIONS TO SURROUNDING TISSUES OF
THE BLACK MATERIAL FREQUENTLY ASSOCIATED WITH THE FUNGUS-
DISEASE OF INDIA.

It must strike even the most casual reader, that the occurrence of these peculiar lumps of black substance in the midst of the

The dark material may be found under three conditions.

tissues referred to in the last chapter, and especially in connection with Specimen V (page 52), is very remarkable; and no one will wonder that it has been found very difficult, or rather impossible, satisfactorily to account for their presence. It will have been observed that these masses have been found, speaking generally, under three conditions: (1), in small completely isolated cavities; (2), in large cavities more or less accurately moulded to their walls; and (3), as broken fragmentary masses lodged in irregular cavities and channels communicating freely with the surface.

As there is less disturbance of the surrounding tissues where the dark masses are found enclosed in minute cysts, they will present fewer complications, and are therefore more instructive than the large tumours described in connection with the last specimen, with all the extensive alterations which had taken place in connection with them; in other words, the significance of the larger masses will become more evident after examination of the smaller ones which are found under less complicated conditions.

Whilst describing specimens of the pale variety,

Isolated granules of the dark material.

Chapter III (Specimen IV, page 27), and Specimens II and III (pp. 49,50) of the dark variety of the disease in the last chapter, attention has been drawn to the fact, that certain of the fat lobules in the subcutaneous tissues had undergone some alteration; whereas other immediately adjoining fat lobules were apparently in the normal state, or only altered to a trifling extent. Some of these altered lobules found in preparations of the dark variety of the disease have contained dark granules. The accompanying wood-cut of a dissection under a low power of a little group of this kind will more clearly convey our meaning. A little of the subcutaneous tissue from over the ankle joint of Specimen II (page 49) was removed and spread out under the dissecting microscope for the purpose of examining a minute dark speck in the midst of what seemed to be normal adipose tissue, and which seemed likely to prove to be the peculiar dark substance found in connection with the malady, enclosed in a capsule. This encysted little mass was found lying be-tween two somewhat hardened, otherwise normal, healthy en-cysted aggregations of fat, as delineated in the engraving (Fig. 7), in which the lining membrane surrounding the dark material is represented as torn open. This capsule was, how-ever, more dense than the cap-sules surrounding the ordinary fat masses, although it resem-

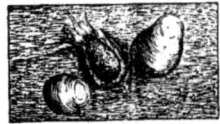

Fig. 7.—Three encysted mass-es of altered adipose and con-nective tissue. The centre one torn open and showing the cha-racteristic black granules. × 6.

bled them in general appearance. Microscopically it consisted of connective tissue, but with a smaller proportion of elastic fibres than those of the normal capsules. It was easily teased out. The material en-closed by the capsule consisted of an aggregation of smooth, black, ova-like particles, each of which was contained in a separate fibrous capsule similar in struc-ture to the general investing capsule, so that the bodies were, although closely aggregated, quite distinct from one another. The black matter could be readily pressed out from the capsules, leaving the latter more or less empty.

Whatever may be the nature of the agent which determined the formation of this minute saccule of dark granules in the midst of saccules of fat cells, it can

scarcely be doubted that it must be essentially identical
in character with the agent which determined the formation of the large nodular masses in the midst of the
bones and areolar tissue of the same preparation—the
darkened material being in the two cases of precisely
similar composition.

There are, moreover, many gradations in the character
and extent of the changes
between the two extremes
just referred to. The ac-
cumulation of granules
may considerably increase
in size and the fibrous en-
velope become stronger
(Fig. 8); this condition
may become more and
more marked, until even-
tually large portions of the
ordinary tissue of a part
become replaced by the
black masses and their tough fibrous receptacles.

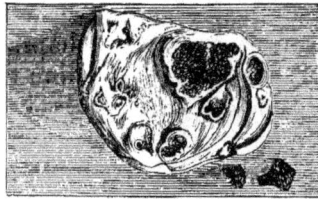

Fig. 8.—A fragment of the affected
tissue from a foot, showing the thickened
fibrous septa forming the cavities, some of
which are seen to contain the black substance: a few particles of the latter are
seen below, out of the cavities.

The physical characters of this peculiar dark substance are, briefly, these : The colour
varies from brownish-yellow to red-
dish-brown and black. The consistence of the different
masses also varies somewhat, apparently according to the
relative proportion of unchanged fatty material associated with it, upon which also the variations in colour
appear to depend. The specific gravity also varies;
generally it may be referred to as being somewhat
greater than water. Some of the lumps, however, sink
almost as readily as a stone when placed in this fluid.
We have never seen examples of the substance that
would float either in spirit or in water.

When placed under the blow-pipe it burns into a
flame, giving off fumes suggestive of
burnt feathers. After being subjected
to this heat for some minutes, a very light dirty-white
ash remains, portions of which under the microscope

*The variations in tint
and the specific gravity
of the dark material.*

*Effect of the applica-
tion of heat—Chemical
characters of the ash.*

present a reticulated semi-cellular aspect. The ash dissolves slightly in water, and the solution yields a strongly alkaline re-action to test paper. The greater portion of what remains undissolved by the water is speedily dissolved by dilute hydrochloric acid, and the solution gives with sulphuric acid the characteristic re-action of a lime compound.

A fragment of bone from the same foot was similarly burnt, and the ash was found to yield very similar re-actions, except, perhaps, that the solution of the ash in water was less alkaline to test paper.

The dark material is insoluble in water and spirit, and only sparingly so in ether, but is almost completely soluble in potash. Weak acids do not materially affect it.

Since these remarks were in type, we have received *Analysis of the black* a note from Mr. C. H. Wood, at *material by Mr. C. H.* *Wood.* present the Officiating Professor of Chemistry at the Medical College, and whose assistance we have already had occasion to acknowledge in this Report, giving a brief account of the result of examinations of fragments of the black substance which he kindly undertook at our request. According to Mr. Wood, the material yielded—

Moisture (by drying at 100° C)	...	...	76·7
Mineral matter	...	...	...	1·4
Organic matter (containing a trace of fat soluble in ether)	...	...	...	21·9

100·0

" In the dry state" 'Mr. Wood writes, "it is quite brittle and may be powdered. The ash is of a red colour from the presence of oxide of iron, but consists chiefly of calcium phosphate. The substance is unaffected by boiling water or acetic acid. Dilute hydrochloric acid gradually extracts a little colour from it, but the alkalis are its only solvents. It forms with potash a brown solution and softens in ammonia undergoing partial disintegration. In its chemical characters this substance somewhat resembles elastic tissue."

The solution of the black material obtained, after subjecting the substance to prolonged ebullition in distilled water, does not yield any characteristic appearance when examined with the spectroscope; nor does a similar solution when treated with sulphuric acid. When, however, some of the material has been dissolved in caustic potash and examined with the spectroscope, it is found that the solution obscures the violet end of the spectrum as far as about the middle of the green, the violet and nearly all the blue being completely absorbed. Blood treated with potash yields a very similar spectrum, but we could not make out the absorption bands of hæmatine in any of the numerous solutions in which the darkened substance had been macerated.

Spectroscopic character of its solutions.

It is the microscopical appearance of this material, however, which presents the most marked peculiarity; that is to say, its microscopical appearance after a more or less prolonged immersion in liquor potassæ. The most satisfactory method of procedure is to crush a lump of the material about the size of a hazel nut, and place it in a test tube with about half an ounce of a strong solution of potash: when set aside for three or four days, it will generally be found that the granular consistence of the substance has disappeared, the fluid has become of a dark color, which subsequently passes into a pale sherry color, and that a small flocculent sediment has subsided in the tube—not more than one-fiftieth, however, of the amount of material introduced. A little of this should be carefully transferred on to a drop of water placed on a glass slide, very gently spread out by means of needles, a covering glass applied and

The microscopical character of the dark material.

the slide examined under a power of from three to five hundred diameters.

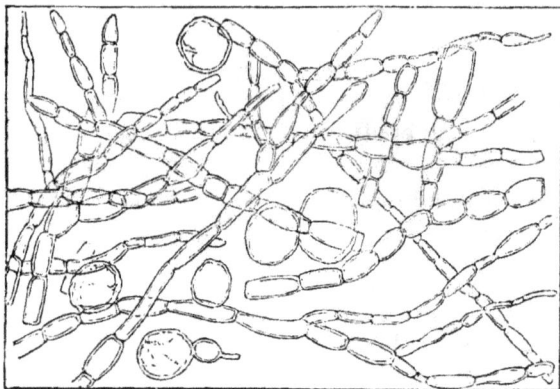

Fig. 9.—Fungoid filaments and capsules obtained after prolonged maceration of the black substance in caustic potash. × 500.

The accompanying wood-cut very accurately represents what will, in all probability, be observed (Fig. 9), *viz.*, numerous branching filaments, septate and perfectly translucent, mixed to a greater or less extent with empty looking cellular bodies. Morphologically, these filaments are not distinguishable from those of fungi, but they do not appear to contain any plasma.

They are capable of withstanding the influence of a large number of powerful re-agents, as the following list will indicate :—

The effect of re-agents on the filaments.

Potash has no destructive influence upon the filaments, or on the capsules associated with them.

Carbolic Acid and Alcohol.—No effect after 15 minutes, nor did the subsequent addition of potash alter the appearance of the preparation.

Bisulphide of Carbon.—No effect.

Benzene.—Filaments were boiled in this fluid for several hours, and also in *chloroform*, without producing any marked change.

Olive Oil and Animal Fat (butter).—Various specimens were boiled in these substances without result, except that, eventually, the filaments became charred owing to the high heat to which the oils had been subjected. Some specimens were subjected to being treated in oil for 12 hours over a water bath.

Tincture of Iodine stains them yellow, and sometimes appears by its reaction to suggest that the tubes and cells are not void of plasma, as they appear to be prior to the addition of the iodine. It never communicates a blue tint to any of these structures, not even when combined with sulphuric acid.

Sulphuric Acid destroys the filaments, so does concentrated hydrochloric acid, perhaps owing to the presence of sulphuric acid in it.

Oxalic Acid also, when concentrated, causes the filaments to disappear.

Carmine.—After prolonged immersion in an ammoniacal solution of this material, the filaments and cells become stained.

Filaments of various fungi, when treated with the foregoing re-agents, were found to manifest pretty much the same properties as the filaments above referred to as having been obtained from the dark substance after maceration in caustic potash.

Occasionally, particles are observed in the field in
<small>Amylaceous particles occasionally found associated with preparations.</small> connection with preparations of the black material, which readily strike a blue, or dark blue, tint on the addition of iodine; but we have not been able to satisfy ourselves that such starchy compounds had not been derived accidentally—from poultices and what not—so that we are not disposed to lay any special stress on the circumstance.

The only other fact which the microscope reveals
<small>The black pigment.</small> worthy of special mention in connection with this dark substance, as far as we have been able to see, is the more or less marked presence of black pigment-particles which may frequently be distin-

guished among the filaments after maceration in the potash solution. These particles sometimes appear as if deposited within the filaments, and occasionally the filaments may be observed to manifest a distinct pigmentary staining; so that, although the alkali may dissolve the greater portion of the pigment in the substance, some of the pigmentary granules remain unaffected, as is the case with the black pigment found in animal tissues generally.

CHAPTER VIII.

CULTIVATIONS OF THE VARIOUS MORBID PRODUCTS OF THE DISEASES.

HAVING now given an account of our investigations into the nature of the changes and degenerations caused by the disease and the characters of their morbid products, we shall next state briefly the results of our attempts at cultivations of these products. In doing this, we shall in some degree depart from the order which we have hitherto followed in the consideration of the different forms of the disease; for it appears advisable to consider those cultivations in which the material experimented with contained distinct fungoid elements, before those in which there was no evidence of the presence of any such bodies.

In undertaking cultivation-experiments of this character, the principal difficulty usually consists, not in selection of ingredients favourable to the growth of the object under observation, but in the isolation of the latter. To follow the growth of a single spore or a speck of plasma may seem a very simple matter to such as have never undertaken such an experiment, but the task is in reality very difficult if the germ experimented upon be given a fair chance of growth—at least as far as light, heat, air, and moisture are concerned. The appliance which we have devised, and for some time adopted, to meet this difficulty, is very simple, and may be constructed by any one desirous of working out for themselves problems of this character. A glance at

the wood-cut will be sufficient to convey a clear conception of its construction. (Fig. 10.)

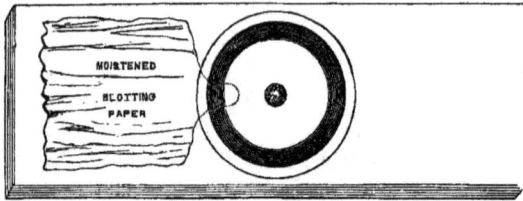

Fig. 10.—A growing-cell adapted for supplying the preparation with moist-air.

It consists of an ordinary glass slide 3″ × 1″, with a
ring of bees' wax (softened by the addition of a little
oil) pressed on its surface towards the middle. Intervening between the wax and slide—clamped by it—is a
narrow slip of blotting-paper; and above the wax a
thin cover-glass is placed with a drop of fluid containing the spore or germ to be watched. The preparation
will now be hermetically sealed except at the spot where
the blotting-paper is inserted, the latter serving as an
excellent channel for the air and moisture necessary to
the perfect growth of the object under cultivation.
There is no danger of dust being introduced, and the
gases which the nutritive fluid may generate can readily escape.

A.—Cultivations of the Black material from the second form of the Madura-Disease.

The materials employed in these experiments were
Cultivations of the obtained from various specimens, and
black matter. consisted in some instances of portions of the black matter which had been discharged
from the tissues previous to the removal of the affected
extremities, and which had been preserved by being simply dried. In other cases the material was obtained
from specimens which had been preserved for longer or
shorter periods in alcohol, glycerine, and other preservative media. The following may serve as examples of
such cultivations and of the results obtained from them.

CULTIVATION I.—Portions of black matter discharg-
A sun-dried specimen
on rice-paste. ed from the foot previous to amputation in a case of the disease, and
which were subsequently dried, were set in some freshly
prepared rice-paste beneath a bell glass. The cultivation was commenced in the month of April.

Forty-eight hours after it had been set, the cultivation was everywhere covered with a dense crop of *Mucor*,
bearing an abundance of ripe, black sporangia. At various points in the paste, patches of a greenish discoloration had appeared; and in one place there was a faint
indication of a pinkish tint present. As, however,
appearances of a similar nature were also present in a
simultaneous cultivation of pure rice-paste, and were
there associated with the occurrence of changes and
developments precisely similar to those here present, the
coloration being, moreover, much more distinctly marked, a fuller description of them is deferred until the
particulars of that cultivation are given. There were,
in addition, several patches of young *Aspergillus* heads
of a white color. During the next few days there was
a rapid increase in the growth of *Mucor*, the loose filaments of which obscured the surface of the paste with
the other fungal elements occurring on it.

Six days after the commencement of the cultivation,
this loose overgrowth was cleared off and a luxuriant
crop of *Aspergillus* was exposed to view. This consisted of two species of the above-mentioned genus—the
first, the common yellow *Aspergillus*; the second, another species, of very frequent occurrence in Calcutta,
in which the heads are of a rich brown colour and the
spores of very minute size. The latter arise from sterigmata, which are not, as in the yellow species, inserted
directly on the globose extremity of the fertile filament,
but are arranged in fours on the broad extremities of
large cuneiform processes intervening between them and
the latter. A dense felt of mycelial filaments and fallen
spores covered the surface of the paste, and on carefully
removing this, the black particles were found, to all
appearance, entirely unaltered.

Immediately around some of them the substance of the paste was of a brownish orange hue, but no peculiar organisms could be found in such places, and there was no evidence of germination or growth of any kind from the black matter. This staining may have been due to a certain amount of solution of the coloring matter of the particles; but even this is very doubtful, as similar staining was frequently observed in cultivations of pure rice-paste to which no black particles had been added. The felt of mycelium having been removed as thoroughly as possible, the specimen was again set aside. It soon became covered anew with yellow and brown *Aspergilli*, together with a smaller regrowth of *Mucor*, whilst patches of *Penicillium glaucum* also began to make their appearance here and there.

Subsequently, one or two patches of dull reddish discoloration appeared, consisting of a granular basis through which colorless mycelial filaments ramified, but they were of the same nature as those which occurred in other instances on pure rice-paste and showed no signs of being in any way organically connected with the black particles. The cultivation was kept under observation for three weeks, and at the close of that time was almost entirely covered with a dense •layer of *Penicillium glaucum*, with a small quantity of *Mucor* still occurring here and there. The black particles showed all their characteristic features under microscopical examination, and afforded no evidences of any attempts at germination nor any signs of vitality on the part of the fungoid elements present in them.

CULTIVATION II.—Contemporaneously with the above cultivation, another was carried out in which a portion of the same rice-paste was set beneath a separate bell glass without the addition of any foreign matter.

Corrective cultivation of pure rice-paste. Development of a pink mould.

This also became rapidly covered with a crop of *Mucor*; ripe fructification, however, appearing not quite so rapidly as in the previous case. The substance of the paste forty-eight hours after the commencement of the experiment was everywhere discolored by dull green patches, whilst here and there minute points of brilliant carmine pink were present. The latter were carefully examined with the following results. The masses of pink matter were mainly composed of a gelatinous basis full of minute particles, and both of these elements were of a bright rosy colour. Where filaments of mycelium penetrated such masses, their contents also were frequently of a similar bright pink, and this coloration of the protoplasm in many cases was not confined to those portions which were absolutely within, or in contact with, the colored material, but continued for some distance farther, rendering the affected filaments very conspicuous, as pink or carmine bands among the surrounding colorless mycelial and bacterial elements, and gradually fading off so as to leave them in their original condition.

The pink coloring was not confined to the living bodies present in the cultivation, but also affected portions of the tissue of the rice grains in the paste. The pink color was confined to the protoplasm of the mycelium, and did not affect the walls of the filaments, for, when the former was made to contract under the influence of re-agents, the latter, which were then more or less widely separated from it, were seen to be perfectly colorless.

These patches of pink color were of a very transitory nature; they had entirely disappeared in forty-eight hours after they were first observed, and there was no recurrence of them afterwards, although the cultivation was kept for several weeks under observation. The *Mucor* never showed such a luxuriance of growth and fructification in this as in the former cultivation, and the paste ultimately became covered with a dense coating of *Penicillium glaucum*, and of a form of *Helminthosporium* with a dark brown mycelium. A few orange-colored stains, like those in Cultivation I, also appeared on the paste, but these showed no special peculiarities on microscopical investigation.

It is needless to repeat the details of numerous other experiments on cultivation of the black masses, as the results were in all cases essentially similar to those described above, and this both where the materials had and had not been subjected to preservation in alcohol or other preservative agents.* The only variations observed concerned the species of common moulds which were developed in different instances, and the relative proportions which the individual species bore to one another in the different cultivations. It may be sufficient to state that in no case did any forms of fungi or other organisms appear in cultivations in which the black material was employed, which did not also occur where rice-paste alone was employed, and that in no instance did any of the fungoid elements of the black matter exhibit the faintest indication of any tendency to germinate. On the contrary, one of the most remarkable features in connection with the cultivation was the extremely persistent and seemingly inert nature of the material, the masses being found to all appearance entirely unaltered in character and contents after weeks of immersion in paste (and at all times of the year), in which the most luxuriant development of fungi had occurred.

General results of cultivation of the black matter in rice-paste.

CULTIVATION III.—Cultivation of the black matter in water.

As the peculiar mould, characteristic of, and peculiar to, the diseased tissues, is stated to have been originally observed in a maceration of a specimen of the disease, we tried numerous experiments with the view of ascertaining whether any such development would occur in the instance of the materials at our disposal. A portion of cancellous bone, containing characteristic black masses, was removed from a foot preserved in spirit and set in water in the month of April. The water was at first, on

---

* When the material had been preserved in spirit, &c., it was always carefully washed and immersed in water for several days before being set in the paste.

several successive days, poured off and renewed with a view to get rid of the spirit, and when this had been, apparently, thoroughly accomplished, the maceration was allowed to go on continuously. The specimen was kept under observation for several weeks. No fungi were developed in connection with it, but an abundance of active and still bacterial elements soon made their appearance, and these, together with some maggots which subsequently aided them, rapidly removed all the soft tissues and oily matter connected with the bone, and left the latter and the masses of black matter behind. The black matter never showed any tendency to germinate or to be altered in any way, and on microscopic examination at the close of the experiment, presented all its characteristic features entirely unchanged.

Results of maceration of the black matter in water.

CULTIVATION IV.—This was precisely similar in its nature to the previous cultivation, and was carried on at the same time of year.

In this case, also, an abundant development of *Bacteria* occurred. The soft tissues of the specimen became gradually disintegrated, and a film of a yellowish color and considerable density formed on the surface of the fluid. This was found to consist of a dense layer of *Bacteria* and granular matter, with innumerable active and encysted specimens of several forms of ciliated infusoria. A few colorless, slender mycelial filaments were also present, and here and there were lumps or concretions of fatty matter of a distinctly pinkish tint. There were, however, no evidences of the presence of any peculiar algoid or fungoid organisms, and the black masses remained seemingly quite unaltered during the entire course of the experiment.

A similar experiment and its results.

Numerous other experiments of a like nature, conpucted at the same and at other seasons of the year, and with materials derived from different specimens obtained from different localities, gave similar negative results.

There was a uniform and entire absence of evidence in favour of the presence of any growth of the elements contained in the black matter or of any other signs of vitality in them, and the only remarkable feature presented by the material in this, as in the former series of experiments, was its extreme persistence and apparent resistance to disintegrative changes.

Absence of evidence of living elements in the black matter.

Whilst, however, these experiments not only entirely failed to demonstrate the existence of any living fungoid organisms in the black matter of the disease, but even seemed to indicate that it did not form a favourable basis for the growth of extrinsic fungi, we have on other occasions frequently observed specimens of the masses become mouldy. This has occurred after the rains have fairly set in, and during periods of very damp weather. At such times there is frequently a development of a white mould on the surface of dried specimens of the material; but as this is due to the growth of the common *Aspergillus* on the surface, and not to any germination of the elements of the substance of the masses, it is obviously a matter of no special importance or interest, save as affording a new example of the varied nature of the substrata on which this ubiquitous mould will occur.

Occasional occurrence of mould on its surface.

B.—*Cultivations of the morbid products of the pale variety of the affection.*

The next series of cultivations regarding which some particulars must be given, are those in which the material experimented with consisted of the roe-like masses and other morbid products and tissues obtained from specimens of the ochroid variety of the disease.

Cultivations of morbid products of the pale variety of the disease.

The cultivations of such materials on rice paste need not be specially alluded to, as they gave results which differed in no essential particulars from those in the experiments with the black matter. Some of the cultivations, or rather macerations in water, however, presented some peculiarities and points of interest.

CULTIVATION V.—Some of the cancellated tissue *Cultivation of material from Specimen No. I.* and oily matter were removed from the bones in a specimen described in the present report as Specimen I (page 15) of the pale variety of the disease, and set in a wide-necked bottle of water beneath a bell-glass. The water was once or twice changed at first in order to get rid of the spirit in which the specimen had been preserved and was then allowed to remain undisturbed. No noteworthy change occurred for sometime. After the lapse of a fortnight, the mouth and neck of the bottle were observed to have become covered with a thin layer of mould, which had also spread over a considerable portion of the surface of the fluid. It did not, however, penetrate beneath the surface and was widely remote from the diseased tissues at the bottom of the bottle. When first observed, the mould was of a whitish and greyish tint, and consisted solely of mycelial filaments without any fructifica-*Mould on the surface of the water.* tion, but subsequently the mycelium gave rise to a crop of poor, partially aborted heads of common *Penicillium* and *Aspergillus*. The bone and fatty matter at the bottom of the fluid remained to all appearance entirely unaltered.

During several weeks no further change was observed, save a gradual evaporation of the water and a proportional spread of the mould downwards over the interior surface of the bottle as the latter became exposed *Appearance of pink coloring:* to the air. The fragments of tissue at the bottom now gradually assumed a distinct pale pink hue, and light flocculi of a similar color could be seen attached to them, loosely adherent to the sides of the bottle beneath the water, or forming a light deposit at the bottom. On examining this cloudy flocculent matter microscopically, it was found to be principally composed of a granular basis, which, whenever in mass, presented a distinct pink tint; whilst even the thinnest flakes of it when examined slightly out of focus were more or less characterised by a similar color. A few mycelial filaments were also present, together with myriads of active *Bacteria* and *Vibriones,* numerous active and encysted *Paramecia,* and a sprinkling of large active *Rotifers.* All these organisms, animal as well as vegetable, were in many instances of a distinct pink color, which was more marked, the larger the mass of the organism affected by it; and, specially bright in some of the *Rotifers.* As time went on, this pink staining continued gradually to increase in intensity, and ultimately the deposit became entirely of a dull brick-red mingled with patches of rosy pink.

Affecting the material, infusoria, rotifers, and fungal elements.

The most marked changes observed by aid of the microscope consisted in a great increase in the amount of mycelial filaments in the deposit. These were found in special abundance in the flocculent patches adhering to the sides of the bottle, and where they were present in abundance, the brightest rosy colour also generally prevailed. Among and attached to the filaments, in many places, numerous large cyst-like bodies were found on carefully teasing out the flocculi (Plate I, Fig. 7.) These were rounded, of diameters ranging on an average from $\frac{1}{250}''$ to $\frac{1}{350}''$, and in many cases were full of roundish or oval spore-like bodies of considerable size. In color, like the filaments with which they were connected, they varied greatly; for, while many were colorless, or exhibited various shades of buff or yellowish, others were of a bright pink or rosy hue. They frequently showed traces of a cellular structure, more or less distinctly. These could, in general, be made out readily by examining the cysts in rather deep focus, so as to bring the profile of their broadest portions into view. The constituent cells of the walls were then clearly brought out, giving rise to an appearance of a looped double outline bounding the mass of the cyst. The cellular structure was also seen to advantage in many cases where rupture of the cyst had

Development of cysts on the mycelium.

occurred, with more or less complete evacuation of the contents. The latter were, like their envelopes, frequently stained of a pink color. The precise nature of the connection of the cysts to the filaments, and their mode of development, could not be thoroughly ascertained, as they were so closely entangled among the meshes and covered by the ramifications of the mycelium as to render it a matter of great difficulty to free them for examination, but it was clearly ascertained in several instances that an organic connection existed between them.

The nature of these bodies was for some time a matter of great doubt and obscurity, but they were ultimately ascertained to be imperfectly developed *Eurotia* of the common yellow *Aspergillus* growing on the sides of the bottle and surface of the fluid. Some of them having been observed in many respects very closely to resemble in structure and form the eurotial structures, which we had frequently obtained on the mycelium of *Aspergillus* when submerged or grown on very moist sub-strata, suggested the renewed examination of the mould on the surface of the water and sides of the bottle—above the fluid in this instance. On doing so, no doubt could remain as to the nature of the submerged bodies. Some of the patches of mould on the sides of the bottle, and which extended from above downwards into the fluid, showed normal yellow specimens of the *Eurotium* of the common yellow *Aspergillus* in their upper portions, and a series of transition forms lower down, until in the submerged parts specimens were present which were precisely similar to the cysts of the deposit, save that none of them were of a pink color, but all colorless or pale yellow (Plate I, Fig. 6.) As, however, the presence and degree of coloring in the cysts below was not a uniform phenomenon, and as other organisms present in the cultivation both at the surface and bottom of the fluid showed a pink tint only in those specimens in the latter situation, this difference did not appear to be of any importance. It certainly could not weigh against

The nature of the cysts— Eurotia.

the numerous points of resemblance or identity in regard to form, size and structure of the cysts, the nature of their contents, and their relations to the filamentous mycelium with which they were connected.

The only question of any importance regarding the submerged specimens related to their development. Were they, and the mycelium bearing them, developed beneath the fluid, or were the submerged flocculi mere fragments of the mould developed above in contact with the air and which had become detached and had subsequently acquired their pink color beneath the fluid? The latter is, perhaps, the more probable of the alternatives; but either mode of development may readily have taken place, as there was an abundance of spores produced by the *Aspergillus* heads originally developed, and these may either have germinated above or at the bottom of the fluid. The spore-like bodies produced within the cysts were peculiar, being unlike those in the *Eurotia* of some other forms of *Aspergillus*, and no asci were observed. They may possibly not have been true spores, but merely abortive asci; as, however, similar bodies may be observed in *Eurotia* developed on other substrata, as will be pointed out subsequently, this is a matter of no special importance in so far as the object of the cultivation in the present instance is concerned.

Questions regarding their development.

The cultivation was kept under observation for several months, but the only further change of any importance which was observed to occur in it was a gradual increase in the depth and intensity of the coloring of the deposit, which ultimately became in great part of a bright vermilion hue. The coloring matter was tested with liquor potassæ at various stages of its development, but in no case did it show any signs of being affected by the re-agent in a manner similar to that exhibited by the coloring matter of the red concretionary particles of the diseased tissues.

Coloring matter not the same as that of the red particles.

With regard to the development of *Aspergillus* in connection with the products of the disease in the above

THE FUNGUS-DISEASE OF INDIA.

cultivation, it may be remarked that species of that genus may very frequently be observed in Calcutta on such materials as skin, cartilage, &c., after the rainy season has set in. We have recently had a striking example of this in regard to one of the commonest species of *Aspergillus*.

Aspergillus develop-ed on animal substances.

The costal cartilages adherent to the skeleton of a dog were observed to present a mouldy aspect, and this on closer examination was found to be dependent on the presence of an abundance of minute white points. Under a low magnifying power these were found to consist of perithecia, presenting the normal features characterising those of *Eurotium*. They were connected with a thin web of white creeping mycelium which formed a net-work over the surface of the cartilage. The perithecia showed the normal cellular structure and were full of roundish or fusiform spores. The perithecia varied considerably in size, ranging from $\frac{1}{470}''$ to $\frac{1}{208}''$ in diameter, and the spores measured on an average $\frac{1}{4166}''$ by $\frac{1}{5000}''$, or when circular $\frac{1}{4166}''$ (*vide* Plate I., Fig. 8). No asci could be detected.

A portion of the cartilage was removed and set in a moist chamber for further examination. Some of the perithecia assumed a yellowish tint, but the majority remained unchanged, and the principal growth observed occurred in the mycelium. The filaments of this became greatly developed, ramifying and anastomosing over the cartilage and forming closely adherent net-works over the surfaces of the perithecia. They presently gave origin to an abundance of erect filaments bearing the ordinary fructification of *Aspergillus*. In many instances these filaments appeared to arise directly from the perithecia, but this was apparently due rather to their origin from adherent mycelial filaments than to the germination of the spores in the interior of the perithecia, or any outgrowth from their walls. The heads of the *Aspergillus* were at first white, and ultimately assumed the bright green tint characteristic of *Aspergillus glaucus*. Spores which had escaped from ruptured perithecia also quickly germinated, and the specimen rapidly became so obscured by a dense growth of mycelium and fructification as to be no longer fit for examination.

Various other macerations of the morbid products of the ochroid variety of the disease were kept under observation during various periods, but in none of them did a development occur as in the case described, nor were any special organisms observed to occur in connection with them which did not equally occur in macerations or other cultivations of other substrata.

Results of other cultivations of the products of the pale variety of the disease.

C.—Cultivations in which the morbid products of the pale variety had been intentionally inoculated with various spores, &c.

Another series of cultivations was conducted with similar materials, but in which these were intentionally inoculated with the conidia and mycelia of various species of fungi. The following may serve as an example of such experiments and of the results occurring in them.

CULTIVATION VI.—Cultivation of inoculated materials. A mass of roe-like bodies, collected from the cavities in Specimen No. III (page 20) of the present report, were immersed in water for several days, the fluid being occasionally changed in order to remove the spirit. It was then set in a moist chamber, and inoculated with some of the black-capsuled *Mucor* and brown and yellow *Aspergilli*, previously described as occurring abundantly in some of the other cultivations. The fungi rapidly grew and spread over the substratum, covering it with a thick crust principally composed of the fructification of the *Aspergilli*—the brown species occurring in considerable excess of the yellow one.

Cultivation in which fungi were purposely introduced.

A month after the inoculation had been performed, this crust was broken up and a layer of bright red matter, varying from rosy pink to strong carmine in color, was found beneath it on the surface of substratum. On microscopic examination, this colored layer was found to be due to a diffused staining of the substratum where the mycelium had penetrated it. Where this had occurred, the material was also softened, but the penetration of the mycelium, the staining and the softening, were all quite superficial, extending only to a very inconsiderable distance beneath the surface of the mass, which elsewhere retained its ordinary characters entirely unaltered. In many instances the fungal filaments and masses of fallen conidia, although embedded in this colored basis, did not participate in the staining, but in others the fungal elements were dyed in all shades from pale pink to bright carmine.

Appearance of a red layer in it.

In some places filaments and growing heads of both the species of *Aspergillus* were found *in situ*, the stems, rounded heads, sterigmata and spores being stained of the brightest carmine, and one or two similarly dyed specimens of *Mucor* filaments and capsules were likewise encountered (Plate I, Figs. 2—5). In the case of the *Aspergilli*, various degrees of staining could be traced among the innumerable heads and conidia present, and a careful determination of the measurements and forms of the latter clearly showed that the rose-colored specimens were mere varieties of the common yellow and brown species along with which they occurred. The coloring was, as usual, confined to the protoplasmic contents of the cells and filaments, whilst the material forming the cell walls was quite colorless. On testing the coloring matter of the substratum and fungi it was found to resemble that of the red concretions, in being partially bleached and rendered brownish by alkalis and generally restored to its orignal condition by the subsequent addition of acids. The re-action of the colored layer was distinctly acid. This red color-

Red Aspergillus

Coloring matter resembled that of the red concretions in its reactions.

ing was not of long duration in the cultivation, only
remaining visible for about a week after its first appearance. The surface of the substratum then became again
covered with a dark-brown coating, principally composed
of the spores of the brown *Aspergillus*, mingled with
a felt of mycelium belonging to that and the yellow
species.

The principal points of interest in this cultivation
were—1st, the demonstration afforded

Both a sexual and
sexual fructification of
Aspergillus liable to become colored.

of the fact that common moulds,
usually occurring on vegetable sub-
stances, found the conditions suitable for their abundant
growth and fructification when cultivated on the material
of the roe-like masses of the degeneration; 2nd, the
developement of red coloring matter in the substratum
and the coincident staining of the fungal elements. It
was specially interesting to obtain colored specimens
of the common conidial fructification of *Aspergillus*
in this cultivation in connection with the occurrence of
similarly colored specimens of the Eurotial or sexual
fructification of the same genus in the experiment previously detailed.

Numerous other similar experiments with inoculated
materials were tried with varying

Results of other simi-
lar experiments.

results. In none, however, was any
development of red coloring observed to occur. The
fungi employed usually grew and fructified freely,
ultimately covering the surface of the substratum. All
the observations agreed in showing that the fungal
elements remained quite superficial, never penetrating
deeply into the mass of the material, and that the
latter was very persistent and remained to all appearance
unaltered during long intervals of time.

(d).—Cultivations in connection with the RED PARTICLES.

Besides the above-mentioned attempts at cultivation
of the black masses, roe-like material

Experiments on cul-
tivation of the red
concretions.

and other morbid products of the
common varieties of the disease, numerous other experi-

ments of a like nature were also carried on in reference to the red concretions. These, however, do not call for any detailed description, as, although carried out at various times, on various substrata, and under very various conditions, they only agreed in showing the entire absence of any development of peculiar organisms and the extremely inert and resistant nature of the concretions. They were never observed to undergo any perceptible change, save a slight alteration of color in some instances, even when kept for weeks under observation.

CHAPTER IX.

LESSONS TO BE DERIVED FROM THESE CULTIVATION EXPERIMENTS.

IT will be evident from the above brief account of the results of our attempts at cultivation of the various morbid products of the disease, that we have entirely failed in obtaining the development of any special species of fungi or other organisms from the latter. The forms which made their appearance in connection with them were only those which are prone to occur indiscriminately on substrata of a most miscellaneous nature, and the only feature characteristic of the specimens developed on these special substrata was the fact that, in some instances, they were stained of a red color. This, however, is a phenomenon not confined to cultivations on such materials—we have observed its occurrence under very various conditions and in very dissimilar media, among others in solutions of choleraic excreta (Plate I, Fig 9)—and, even had it been so, the circumstance would have been of no value as an indication of specific peculiarities in the colored organisms.

No peculiar species of vegetable organisms developed in cultivations of the various morbid materials.

Any one who has studied the varied developments of common moulds, or other low vegetable organisms, must be well aware that mere color, independent of structural peculiarities, is as untrustworthy a basis for the determination of specificity in regard to them as it is in regard to higher organisms. It may, however, be argued that, allowing that our experiments showed no evidence of the presence of any peculiar specific forms in the products of the disease, it is sufficient that varieties characterised by certain features, such as color, were developed. It may be affirmed that the presence of peculiar colors implies a difference of con-

Mere color insufficient to determine specificity.

stitution, and a corresponding difference of properties in the colored varieties, as compared with the ordinary ones, and that the peculiarity of coloring in the varieties with which we are at present concerned coincides with the peculiar property of inducing the 'Madura Disease.'

We believe, however, that there are points in our observations which negative any such belief, and which justify us in ascribing the peculiarities of coloring to the nature of the substratum, and not to that of any peculiar varieties of organisms present, or assumed to be present in it. In one experiment in which the color was peculiarly well marked, it was not confined to any special vegetable forms, nor even to vegetable organisms, but appeared equally in the ciliate infusoria and *Rotifers;* whilst, in another cultivation, various species of fungi artificially introduced into the morbid materials became equally highly colored whilst growing in and on them. It can hardly be supposed that the colored varieties of *Rotifers* had any connection with the morbid products of the disease, save occurring in the water along with them, and possibly deriving their nourishment from them.

Peculiarities of coloring in the present instance ascribable to nature of substratum.

As to the colored fungi of the other cultivation, it is manifest that their peculiarities were dependent on the conditions under which they were developed or to which they were subjected, for the species affected were not only among the commonest forms of moulds, but only acquired their peculiar characters as to color when artificially exposed to the influences of the substratum. It would certainly be unwarrantable to assume that varieties arising in such a way under the influence of certain substrata are necessarily endowed with the power of reproducing similar materials elsewhere.

The fact that the coloring matter present in one of the cultivations was identical in its reactions (with acids and alkalis) with the red coloring matter of the concretions, also points to its dependence on the chemical

Pink coloring not peculiar to fungi developed in connection with the disease-products.

composition of the morbid material, and not to any
inherent special property of the fungal elements acci-
dentally or wilfully developed in association with it.
Moreover, as was observed in the case of the cultivation
of rice-paste forming the second in the series of cultivations here described, and as we have frequently observed
in other instances, pink coloration of the elements of
various moulds is by no means an uncommon phenomenon in this country, and it is one which is assuredly
not confined to cultivations connected with the morbid
products of this or any other disease—indeed, we have
seen it to develop on a dish of drying crystals of lactate
of lime, far removed from the place where these cultivation-experiments were being conducted; so that the
mere occurrence of it in connection with the affection
cannot be regarded as affording any satisfactory evidence
in favour of the dependence of the disease on a peculiar
species, or even on peculiar varieties of fungi.

It appears to us that the original observations on the
occurrence of red colored fungi in
connection with the products of the
disease, point very forcibly in the
same direction as the results of the present cultivations,
and indicate that, whatever the nature of the organisms
observed may have been—whether they belonged to
peculiar genera, or species, or not—they were quite unconnected with the fungoid elements of these products.
It is a remarkable fact that in some instances the
colored moulds were observed, as in our cultivations, in
connection with the products of the pale variety of the
disease, that is, in connection with materials in which
the presence of fungoid elements has never been demonstrated. Moreover, they showed no unequivocal
evidences of specific identity in the different cases; at
all events, in so far as descriptions and illustrations go,
we fail to see that they did so; more than all, they
occurred indifferently as developments in cultivations
where the materials had been subjected to prolonged
preservation in spirit, and in others in which no preservative agent had been employed.

Original observations on this point agree with later experiments.

It has been denied that there is any evidence that spores, or other fungal elements, may not retain their vitality and power of germination in spite of prolonged exposure to the influence of alcohol. In spite of the weight justly attached to the opinion of those holding such ¦views, we would enquire whether there be any evidence showing that they are endowed with any such faculty ? We are not aware of any ; and although by no means wishing to found any sweeping generalisations on limited data, we can only state that the results of our own observations and experiments have been directly opposed to the assumption of the actual existence of such a resisting power.

Effects of alcohol on the vitality of fungal elements.

In connection with the cultivations described in the present report, we have tried numerous careful experiments on the effects of alcohol on the spores and mycelium of fungi, and have never observed such bodies show any signs of having retained their vitality after even very short exposure to the re-agent. In regard to cultivations of the morbid products of the disease, Mr. Berkeley's experience is strongly in support of this, for he states that he entirely failed in obtaining any development from the preserved specimens which were submitted to him, and only obtained a growth of pink mould when working, not with the original morbid materials, but with rice-paste on which similarly colored fungi had previously occurred in Bombay.

Taking everything into consideration, it appears to us that all that has yet been shown by means of cultivations is, that fungi and other organisms developed in connectionwith the morbid products of the 'Madura Disease,' occasionally present themselves in pink or red colored varieties ; and that this coloring is due to the nature of the material, and not to any specific properties in the organisms. The phenomenon, therefore, is one which cannot be cited as a proof of the fungal origin of the disease, or of the presence of fungal elements in materials such as those of the pale variety of the disease, affording no other evidences of their existence.

Pink coloring of the fungi no proof of the fungal origin of the disease.

CHAPTER X.

CONCLUSIONS.

IT now only remains for us to summarise the principal points in connection with the peculiar affection of the feet and hands which we have referred to in detail in the preceding pages. It has been seen that the disease appears in two principal forms; that the lesions produced, the particular tissues affected, and the general course of the disease present much in common; but that the morbid products, whether examined chemically or microscopically, are found to be most dissimilar.

In the pale variety this product is for the most part

Nature of the morbid products. of a fatty nature, abounding in many of the various modifications of fat known to pathologists; whereas in the dark variety, the fatty matter forms a far less prominent feature in some cases; indeed, the dark material may often be referred to as being almost completely devoid of fat—at all events it must have undergone such extensive changes as to be no longer recognisable as such.

It is extremely difficult to account for the discre-

Is the dark variety an earlier stage of the pale? pancy in the composition of the morbid products of the disease. The inference that the pale is a later stage of the dark variety of the affection, as advocated by Dr. Vandyke Carter, is, in our opinion, untenable from the fact that, as has been shown on a previous page, the progress of the disease may, in some cases, be traced through all its stages in a single specimen, just as in a tuberculised lung areas may often be distinguished presenting the most recent deposits of tubercle in the midst of tissue far advanced in the degeneration. In specimen III (page 20) for example, the various steps in the degenerative process could be followed with the greatest ease. Well defined areas could be seen in the midst of, apparently, healthy connective and fatty tissues, and the various stages of the process, trifling consolidation of defined areas of tissue, slight discoloration, nests of roe-like bodies associated or not with crystalline formations, and other changes, could be readily identified, but without any indication of the previous existence of the black substance.

On the other hand we have seen specimens of the dark variety in such a recent stage of the development of the malady, as to negative any idea of its being a later stage of the pale; the dark granules, not larger than grains of gunpowder, being deposited here and there among the tissues; the only concomitant alterations of the part being slight hardening and trifling discoloration of isolated lobules in the subcutaneous tissue. In one case (Specimen II, pages 95 and 99), we were able to trace what appeared to us to be the progressive stages, in this variety also, of the malady—from the yellowish-brown ceruminous nodule, to the almost perfect black granular lump.

The various stages in the progress of the Dark variety.

It is nevertheless quite possible, and indeed probable, judging from the great similarity in the lesions produced, the course pursued by the disease, and its duration in the two forms, that the original cause may be very closely allied if not identical. Pathology has not yet progressed sufficiently to be able to determine why it is that certain degenerations will take very different courses in different persons; nor is the science sufficiently advanced to enable us to refer definitely to the direct cause of almost any single degenerative process. For the most part our etiological conceptions are hypothetical. Consequently we are no further behind in our knowledge of the etiology of this comparatively new disease than we are with reference to the causation of the various cancerous and other morbid processes which have been known for centuries.

The cause of both not improbably identical.

But do we know *more* as to the cause of this disease than we do of most others? Certainly the forms under which the disease manifests itself are in many ways different from those ordinarily met with: it is characterised by being localis-

Clinical characteristics of the affection.

ed to certain districts, and by the fact that only certain parts of the body, as far as we at present know, are liable to be affected; and more than all, the morbid product of one, or rather of two, of its varieties, the black and the pink, are so peculiar, as to enable it to be distinguished at once from all other affections. But that these peculiarities should of themselves be sufficient ground for forming any conclusions with reference to the *cause* of the affection, is not supported by the observations which we have made.

The reader of the foregoing chapters will have observed that three of the peculiar morbid products described as various stages in the development of a peculiar fungus, the assumed cause of the disease, have been very carefully investigated, *viz.*, the roe-like bodies, the pink particles, and the black masses.

The real nature of the roe-like and pink particles, and the black masses.

The first of these we have shown to be fat in various modified forms ; the second were found to be pigmented concretions—not the slightest trace of a fungus or of other vegetable organisims being present in either; and the third we have shown to consist of degenerated tissue, mixed to a greater or less extent with black pigment and fungoid filaments. To account for the presence of the two latter ingredients is in reality the most difficult problem connected with the affection.

As regards the actual lesions produced in the tissues, it will have been observed that neither of these two latter ingredients are essential, seeing that, with the exception of the physical characters of the morbid products, no marked distinction exists between the pale and the black varieties. Similar tissues are affected in both, the cavities and channels are alike, and the similarity extends even to the peculiar mammillated orifices by which these open on the surface. These circumstances of themselves absolutely negative, in our opinion, the view that anything which may be found in connection with one variety, and not in connection with the other, can be referred to as the specific cause of either. Why

No etiological significance can be attributed to the presence of pigment and filaments in the dark variety.

these morbid substances should present these anomalies is a totally different question, and one which is not within our province to discuss.

The occurrence of pigmentary deposits in animal tissues is by no means a rare circumstance. Our knowledge as to whence the pigment is derived is not yet very exact, but it is generally believed to be derived from the blood. Its behaviour under the influence of re-agents is, however, well known, and we have found that the pigment in the dark substance, when treated with re-agents, manifests properties similar to those of ordinary pigment. The presence of iron in the pigmented substance of the Madura-disease, which both Mr. Wood's analysis and our own revealed, is a significant fact, seeing that iron is a constant component of black pigment, a circumstance which, in our opinion, points almost unequivocally to the fact that the pigmented substance under consideration originates from the same material as the pigmentary deposits ordinarily met with in animal tissues.

Probable nature and source of the pigment.

We have already given full particulars regarding the microscopical and chemical properties of the fungoid elements associated with the pigment; they resist the action of weak acids and strong alkalis, and manifest all the properties of ordinary fungal forms except vitality; and we believe that it will be generally conceded that it has been shown that on no single occasion has any one been able to coax the fungoid elements in this substance to germinate, much less to develop anything approaching to mature fruit; hence any propositions which may have been advanced with regard to the causation of the Madura-disease on the grounds that a new or peculiar fungus has been developed from the morbid products amongst the tissue are, apparently, without good foundation and must be carefully reconsidered in the light of the facts now adduced. It is for botanists to decide whether the ' *Chionyphe Carteri* ' is what is termed a "good species" or not; all we have to do with it is restricted to its purely pathological significance, and, in connection with that, we

The fungoid elements in the dark substance not genetically connected with 'Chionyphe Carteri.'

unhesitatingly express our convictions, that not only does it not cause the disease, but that it cannot be developed from the fungoid elements contained in the morbid product.

Although we have failed in inducing these fungoid

The filaments and capsules are probably vegetations.

elements to grow, it does not follow on that account that they are not, and never have been, vitalised. It is true that a great many purely physical products are found which so closely resemble those which have been moulded under the influence of vitality as not to be distinguishable, or only distinguishable with difficulty; such, for example, as the concretions of Mr. Rainey—the *calcospherites* of Professor Harting—the *myeline* of Virchow, and the amylaceous corpuscles known to all microscopists; still, the optical and physical characters of the filaments and capsules seem to us to agree so perfectly with what we have seen in undoubted fungi, that we look upon them as such until the contrary can be demonstrated.

To account for their presence in the tissues—deeply

Whence are the fungoid elements derived?

imbedded and far removed from anything that could suggest the existence of a channel of communication between the spot and the exterior for any such immobile object as a spore, is most puzzling. The supposition that a sporule had managed to insinuate itself by means of some natural, or artificially produced pore, is untenable from the simple fact that perfectly independent *foci* of the affection may be distinguished—so distinctly defined as to necessitate the inference that each localised pigmentary deposit had derived its origin from the introduction (through the cutaneous tissues) into that particular part of a foreign body capable of germinating.

To us it appears much more reasonable to infer that localised spots in the tissues undergo a degenerative change into a substance *peculiarly* adapted to the development of filamentous growths. We ourselves have shown, and it has been shown by others, that under certain conditions—the principal being the absence of vitality, or vitality greatly depressed—every tissue in the body is capable of giving rise to the abundant development of complex organisms.

We reproduce a figure (Fig. 11) of some of the
Experiments show-
ing that fungal forms
invariably appear un-
der favourable circum-
stances in non-living
tissues.
leading forms of these growths. for
convenience of reference from a report
which we submitted last year bearing
on this matter, as we have since that
period undertaken several experiments of a like nature
and which have a very direct bearing on the point now
under consideration. The object of the experiments was
to ascertain whether, by interfering with the vascular
supply of certain tissues and organs of the body of an
animal without injuring the isolated tissue, we should
be able within the course of some hours to detect
organisms in those parts in the same manner as we had
been able to do when an animal had been killed under
chloroform and set aside in a warm place.* We found

---

* In connection with this subject, the question naturally presents itself as to the
degree in which results of this nature are influenced by the conditions of the locality
where the experiments are carried out—whether the results which are obtained under
the influence of the temperature of a tropical climate are likely to occur in temperate
localities with lower temperatures. We believe that they are, and this on the ground
of the following experiment:—

Two men were executed in the Presidency Jail in the month of December 1874.
The bodies were removed to the dead-house immediately after having remained
suspended for the prescribed period. The following statement shows the temperatures
registered at various intervals during the following 24 hours by thermometers
inserted into the substance of the liver and the muscles of the thigh in both bodies
compared with the coincident atmospheric temperature.

Body.	Time after death.	TEMPERATURE.			
		Liver.	Thigh.	Air.	
No. 1 ...	1 hour ...	93°5	88°	62°	Body on a lead-covered table.
	4·5 ,,	91°9	86°5	67°	
	8 ,,	87°0	82°0	68°5	
	15 ,,	84°0	74°0	64°5	
	24 ,,	76°0	69°0	59°	
No. 2 ...	1 hour ...	95°	91°	62°	Body on a wooden table.
	4·5 ,,	92°	86°	67°	
	8 ,,	87°	81°	68°5	
	15 ,,	84°	74°	64°5	
	24 ,,	76°	69°	59°	A

The loss of temperature is so gradual even when the external temperature is moderate,
that in so far as conditions of temperature are concerned, the body, save in exceptional
cases, must, for many hours after death, itself provide a suitable temperature for the
rapid development of organisms.

that such was the result, and that a kidney, for example, when carefully ligatured without interfering with its position in the abdomen, would be found after some

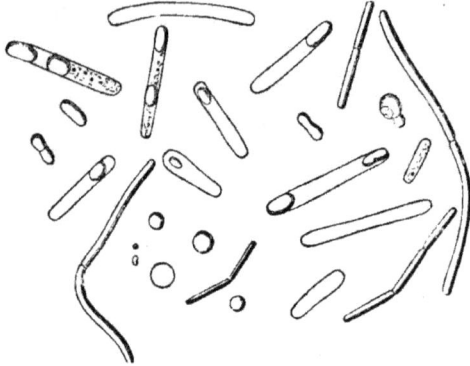

Fig. 11.—Organisms found in the tissues of *healthy* animals a few hours after death. × 1,500.

hours to contain precisely similar organisms ; whereas the other kidney—whose circulation had not been interfered with—contained no trace of any vegetation whatever.

Taking everything into consideration, it seems probable to us that some local degeneration takes place in the Madura-disease, giving rise to a product which is, in one of its varieties, peculiarly adapted to the development of vegetable organisms. All microscopists know how frequently the most trifling alteration in the composition of a nutritive medium decides the advent of peculiar growths.

CALCUTTA, }
September 1875. }

INDEX.

A.

F.

N.

Ebenfalls im SEVERUS Verlag erhältlich:

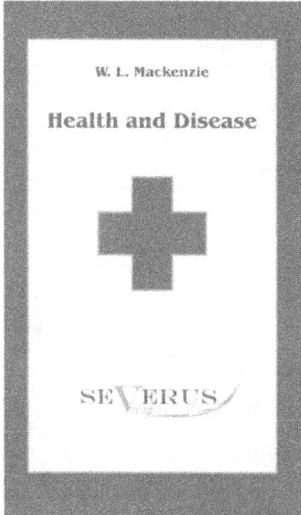

William Leslie Mackenzie
Health and Disease
SEVERUS 2011/ 256 S./ 39,50 Euro
ISBN 978-3-86347-120-0

"The science of public health administration has had no abler or more attractive exponent than Dr Mackenzie. He adds to a thorough grasp of the problems an illuminating style, and an arresting manner of treating a subject often dull and sometimes unsavoury." –Economist

With a near-literary style, William L. Mackenzie (1862-1935) guides the reader through an examination of common diseases, their sources and their prevention. Defining "health" as "a mere working concept, an ideal", he offers a view on the changing health awareness of early 20th century society.

www.severus-verlag.de

Bisher im SEVERUS Verlag erschienen:

Achelis. Th. Die Entwicklung der Ehe * Die Religionen der Naturvölker im Umriß, Reihe ReligioSus Band V * **Andreas-Salomé, Lou** Rainer Maria Rilke * **Arenz, Karl** Die Entdeckungsreisen in Nord- und Mittelafrika von Richardson, Overweg, Barth und Vogel * **Aretz, Gertrude (Hrsg)** Napoleon I - Briefe an Frauen * **Ashburn, P.M** The ranks of death. A Medical History of the Conquest of America * **Avenarius, Richard** Kritik der reinen Erfahrung * Kritik der reinen Erfahrung, Zweiter Teil * **Beneke, Otto** Von unehrlichen Leuten: Kulturhistorische Studien und Geschichten aus vergangenen Tagen deutscher Gewerbe und Dienste * **Berneker, Erich** Graf Leo Tolstoi * **Bernstorff, Graf Johann Heinrich** Erinnerungen und Briefe * **Bie, Oscar** Franz Schubert - Sein Leben und sein Werk * **Binder, Julius** Grundlegung zur Rechtsphilosophie. Mit einem Extratext zur Rechtsphilosophie Hegels * **Bliedner, Arno** Schiller. Eine pädagogische Studie * **Birt, Theodor** Frauen der Antike * **Blümner, Hugo** Fahrendes Volk im Altertum * **Boos, Heinrich** Geschichte der Freimaurerei. Ein Beitrag zur Kultur- und Literatur-Geschichte des 18. Jahrhunderts * **Brahm, Otto** Das deutsche Ritterdrama des achtzehnten Jahrhunderts: Studien über Joseph August von Törring, seine Vorgänger und Nachfolger * **Brandes, Georg** Moderne Geister: Literarische Bildnisse aus dem 19. Jahrhundert. * **Braun, Lily** Lebenssucher * **Braun, Ferdinand** Drahtlose Telegraphie durch Wasser und Luft * **Brunnemann, Karl** Maximilian Robespierre - Ein Lebensbild nach zum Teil noch unbenutzten Quellen * **Büdinger, Max** Don Carlos Haft und Tod insbesondere nach den Auffassungen seiner Familie * **Burkamp, Wilhelm** Wirklichkeit und Sinn. Die objektive Gewordenheit des Sinns in der sinnfreien Wirklichkeit * **Caemmerer, Rudolf Karl Fritz Die** Entwicklung der strategischen Wissenschaft im 19. Jahrhundert * **Casper, Johann Ludwig** Handbuch der gerichtlich-medizinischen Leichen-Diagnostik: Thanatologischer Teil, Bd. 1 * Bd. 2 * **Cronau, Rudolf** Drei Jahrhunderte deutschen Lebens in Amerika. Eine Geschichte der Deutschen in den Vereinigten Staaten * **Cunow, Heinrich** Geschichte und Kultur des Inkareiches * **Cushing, Harvey** The life of Sir William Osler, Volume 1 * The life of Sir William Osler, Volume 2 * **Dahlke, Paul** Buddhismus als Religion und Moral, Reihe ReligioSus Band IV * **Dühren, Eugen** Der Marquis de Sade und seine Zeit. in Beitrag zur Kultur- und Sittengeschichte des 18. Jahrhunderts. Mit besonderer Beziehung auf die Lehre von der Psychopathia Sexualis * **Eckstein, Friedrich** Alte, unnennbare Tage. Erinnerungen aus siebzig Lehr- und Wanderjahren * Erinnerungen an Anton Bruckner * **Eiselsberg, Anton Freiherr von** Lebensweg eines Chirurgen * **Eloesser, Arthur** Thomas Mann - sein Leben und Werk * **Elsenhans, Theodor** Fries und Kant. Ein Beitrag zur Geschichte und zur systematischen Grundlegung der Erkenntnistheorie. * **Engel, Eduard** Shakespeare * Lord Byron. Eine Autobiographie nach Tagebüchern und Briefen. * **Ewald, Oscar** Nietzsches Lehre in ihren Grundbegriffen * Die französische Aufklärungsphilosophie * **Ferenczi, Sandor** Hysterie und Pathoneurosen * **Fichte, Immanuel Hermann** Die Idee der Persönlichkeit und der individuellen Fortdauer * **Fourier, Jean Baptiste Joseph Baron** Die Auflösung der bestimmten Gleichungen * **Frazer, James George** Totemism and Exogamy. A Treatise on Certain Early Forms of Superstition and Society * **Frey, Adolf** Albrecht von Haller und seine Bedeutung für die deutsche Literatur * **Frimmel, Theodor von** Beethoven Studien I. Beethovens äußere Erscheinung * Beethoven Studien II. Bausteine zu einer Lebensgeschichte des Meisters * **Fülleborn, Friedrich** Über eine medizinische Studienreise nach Panama, Westindien und den Vereinigten Staaten * **Gmelin, Johann Georg** Quousque? Beiträge zur soziologischen Rechtfindung * **Goette, Alexander** Holbeins Totentanz und seine Vorbilder * **Goldstein, Eugen** Canalstrahlen * **Graebner, Fritz** Das Weltbild der Primitiven: Eine Untersuchung der Urformen weltanschaulichen Denkens bei Naturvölkern * **Griesinger, Wilhelm** Handbuch der speciellen Pathologie und Therapie: Infectionskrankheiten * **Griesser, Luitpold** Nietzsche und Wagner - neue Beiträge zur Geschichte und Psychologie ihrer Freundschaft * **Hanstein, Adalbert von** Die Frauen in der Geschichte des Deutschen Geisteslebens des 18. und 19. Jahrhunderts * **Hartmann, Franz** Die Medizin des Theophrastus Paracelsus von Hohenheim * **Heller, August** Geschichte der Physik von Aristoteles bis auf die neueste Zeit. Bd. 1: Von Aristoteles bis Galilei * **Helmholtz, Hermann von** Reden und Vorträge, Bd. 1 * Reden und Vorträge, Bd. 2 * **Henker, Otto** Einführung in die Brillenlehre * **Henne am Rhyn, Otto** Aus Loge und Welt: Freimaurerische und kulturgeschichtliche Aufsätze * **Jahn, Ulrich** Die deutschen Opfergebräuche bei Ackerbau und Viehzucht. Ein Beitrag zur Deutschen Mythologie und Altertumskunde * **Kalkoff, Paul** Ulrich von Hutten und die Reformation. Eine kritische Geschichte seiner wichtigsten Lebenszeit und der Entscheidungsjahre der Reformation (1517 - 1523), Reihe ReligioSus Band I * **Kaufmann, Max** Heines Liebesleben * **Kautsky, Karl** Terrorismus und Kommunismus: Ein Beitrag zur Naturgeschichte der Revolution * **Kerschensteiner, Georg** Theorie der Bildung * **Kotelmann, Ludwig** Gesundheitspflege im Mittelalter. Kulturgeschichtliche Studien nach Predigten des 13., 14. und 15. Jahrhunderts * **Klein, Wilhelm** Geschichte der Griechischen Kunst - Erster Band: Die Griechische Kunst bis Myron * **Krömeke, Franz** Friedrich Wilhelm Sertürner - Entdecker des Morphiums * **Külz, Ludwig** Tropenarzt im afrikanischen Busch * **Leimbach, Karl Alexander** Untersuchungen über die verschiedenen Moralsysteme * **Liliencron, Rochus von / Müllenhoff, Karl** Zur Runenlehre. Zwei Abhandlungen * **Mach, Ernst** Die Principien der Wärmelehre * **Mackenzie, William Leslie** Health and Disease * **Maurer, Konrad** Island von seiner ersten Entdeckung bis zum Untergange des Freistaats * **Mausbach, Joseph** Die Ethik des heiligen Augustinus. Erster Band: Die sittliche Ordnung und ihre Grundlagen * **Mauthner, Fritz** Die drei Bilder der Welt - ein sprachkritischer Versuch * **Meissner, Franz Hermann** Arnold Böcklin * **Meyer, Elard Hugo** Indogermanische Mythen, Bd. 1: Gandharven-Kentauren * **Müller, Adam** Versuche einer neuen Theorie des Geldes * **Müller, Conrad Alexander** von Humboldt und das Preußische Königshaus. Briefe aus den Jahren 1835-1857 * **Naumann, Friedrich** Freiheitskämpfe * **Oettingen, Arthur von** Die Schule der Physik * **Ossipow, Nikolai** Tolstois Kindheitserinnerungen. Ein Beitrag zu Freuds Libidotheorie * **Ostwald, Wilhelm** Erfinder und Entdecker * **Peters, Carl** Die deutsche Emin-Pascha-Expedition * **Poetter, Friedrich Christoph** Logik * **Popken, Minna** Im Kampf um die Welt des Lichts. Lebenserinnerungen und Bekenntnisse einer Ärztin * **Prutz, Hans** Neue Studien zur Geschichte der Jungfrau von Orléans * **Rank, Otto** Psychoanalytische Beiträge zur Mythenforschung. Gesammelte Studien aus den Jahren 1912 bis 1914. * **Ree, Paul Johannes** Peter Candid * **Rohr, Moritz von** Joseph Fraunhofers Leben, Leistungen und Wirksamkeit * **Rubinstein, Susanna** Ein individualistischer Pessimist: Beitrag zur Würdigung Philipp Mainländers * Eine Trias von Willensmetaphysikern: Populär-philosophische Essays * **Sachs, Eva** Die fünf platonischen Körper: Zur Geschichte der Mathematik und der Elementenlehre Platons und der Pythagoreer * **Scheidemann, Philipp** Memoiren eines Sozialdemokraten, Erster Band * Memoiren eines Sozialdemokraten, Zweiter Band * **Schleich, Carl Ludwig** Erinnerungen an Strindberg nebst Nachrufen für Ehrlich und von Bergmann * Das Ich und die Dämonien * **Schlösser, Rudolf** Rameaus Neffe - Studien und Untersuchungen zur Einführung in Goethes Übersetzung des Diderotschen Dialogs * **Schweitzer, Christoph** Reise nach Java und Ceylon (1675-1682). Reisebeschreibungen von deutschen Beamten und Kriegsleuten im Dienst der niederländischen West- und Ostindischen Kompagnien 1602 - 1797. * **Schweitzer, Philipp** Island - Land und Leute * **Sommerlad, Theo** Die soziale Wirksamkeit der Hohenzollern * **Stein, Heinrich von** Giordano Bruno. Gedanken über seine Lehre und sein Leben * **Strache, Hans** Der Eklektizismus des Antiochus von Askalon * **Sulger-Gebing, Emil** Goethe und Dante * **Thiersch, Hermann** Ludwig I von Bayern und die Georgia Augusta * Pro Samothrake * **Tyndall, John** Die Wärme betrachtet als eine Art der Bewegung, Bd. 1 * Die Wärme betrachtet als eine Art der Bewegung, Bd. 2 * **Virchow, Rudolf** Vier Reden über Leben und Kranksein * **Vollmann, Franz** Über das Verhältnis der späteren Stoa zur Sklaverei im römischen Reiche * **Volkmer, Franz** Das Verhältnis von Geist und Körper im Menschen (Seele und Leib) nach Cartesius * **Wachsmuth, Curt** Das alte Griechenland im neuen * **Weber, Paul** Beiträge zu Dürers Weltanschauung * **Wecklein, Nikolaus** Textkritische Studien zu den griechischen Tragikern * **Weinhold, Karl** Die heidnische Totenbestattung in Deutschland * **Wellhausen, Julius** Israelitische und Jüdische Geschichte, Reihe ReligioSus Band VI ***Wellmann, Max** Die pneumatische Schule bis auf Archigenes - in ihrer Entwickelung dargestellt * **Wernher, Adolf** Die Bestattung der Toten in Bezug auf Hygiene, geschichtliche Entwicklung und gesetzliche Bestimmungen * **Weygandt, Wilhelm** Abnorme Charaktere in der dramatischen Literatur. Shakespeare - Goethe - Ibsen - Gerhart Hauptmann * **Wlassak, Moriz** Zum römischen Provinzialprozeß * **Wulffen, Erich** Kriminalpädagogik: Ein Erziehungsbuch * **Wundt, Wilhelm** Reden und Aufsätze * **Zallinger, Otto** Die Ringgaben bei der Heirat und das Zusammengeben im mittelalterlich-deutschem Recht * **Zoozmann, Richard** Hans Sachs und die Reformation - In Gedichten und Prosastücken, Reihe ReligioSus Band III